MIX
Papier aus verantwortungsvollen Quellen
Paper from responsible sources
FSC® C105338

Mennatallah Ahmed Ismail Ali

A new approach in Type 2 diabetes mellitus treatment

Evaluation of the beneficial effect of L-cysteine in the treatment of type 2 diabetes mellitus

Anchor Academic Publishing

Ali, Mennatallah Ahmed Ismail: A new approach in Type 2 diabetes mellitus treatment: Evaluation of the beneficial effect of L-cysteine in the treatment of type 2 diabetes mellitus. Hamburg, Anchor Academic Publishing 2015

Buch-ISBN: 978-3-95489-353-9
PDF-eBook-ISBN: 978-3-95489-853-4
Druck/Herstellung: Anchor Academic Publishing, Hamburg, 2015

Bibliografische Information der Deutschen Nationalbibliothek:
Die Deutsche Nationalbibliothek verzeichnet diese Publikation in der Deutschen Nationalbibliografie; detaillierte bibliografische Daten sind im Internet über http://dnb.d-nb.de abrufbar.

Bibliographical Information of the German National Library:
The German National Library lists this publication in the German National Bibliography. Detailed bibliographic data can be found at: http://dnb.d-nb.de

All rights reserved. This publication may not be reproduced, stored in a retrieval system or transmitted, in any form or by any means, electronic, mechanical, photocopying, recording or otherwise, without the prior permission of the publishers.

Das Werk einschließlich aller seiner Teile ist urheberrechtlich geschützt. Jede Verwertung außerhalb der Grenzen des Urheberrechtsgesetzes ist ohne Zustimmung des Verlages unzulässig und strafbar. Dies gilt insbesondere für Vervielfältigungen, Übersetzungen, Mikroverfilmungen und die Einspeicherung und Bearbeitung in elektronischen Systemen.

Die Wiedergabe von Gebrauchsnamen, Handelsnamen, Warenbezeichnungen usw. in diesem Werk berechtigt auch ohne besondere Kennzeichnung nicht zu der Annahme, dass solche Namen im Sinne der Warenzeichen- und Markenschutz-Gesetzgebung als frei zu betrachten wären und daher von jedermann benutzt werden dürften.

Die Informationen in diesem Werk wurden mit Sorgfalt erarbeitet. Dennoch können Fehler nicht vollständig ausgeschlossen werden und die Diplomica Verlag GmbH, die Autoren oder Übersetzer übernehmen keine juristische Verantwortung oder irgendeine Haftung für evtl. verbliebene fehlerhafte Angaben und deren Folgen.

Alle Rechte vorbehalten

© Anchor Academic Publishing, Imprint der Diplomica Verlag GmbH
Hermannstal 119k, 22119 Hamburg
http://www.diplomica-verlag.de, Hamburg 2015
Printed in Germany

LIST OF CONTENTS

Chapter	Page
LIST OF TABLES	ii
LIST OF FIGURES	iv
LIST OF ABBREVIATIONS	vii
I. INTRODUCTION	1
II. AIM OF THE WORK	67
III. MATERIALS AND METHODS	68
IV. RESULTS	97
V. DISCUSSION	161
VI. CONCLUSIONS AND RECOMMENDATIONS	187
VII. SUMMARY	190
VIII. REFERENCES	195

LIST OF TABLES

Table		Page
(1)	Effect of STZ-induced type 2 diabetes on fasting serum glucose, fasting serum insulin and HOMA-IR in male albino rats	103
(2)	Effect of STZ-induced type 2 diabetes on lipid profile in male albino rats	105
(3)	Effect of STZ-induced type 2 diabetes on oxidative stress parameters in male albino rats	108
(4)	Effect of STZ-induced type 2 diabetes on inflammatory parameters in male albino rats	110
(5)	Effect of treatment with the studied drugs for 2 weeks on fasting serum glucose in male albino rats (mg/dl)	113
(6)	Effect of treatment with the studied drugs for 2 weeks on fasting serum insulin in male albino rats (ng/ml)	116
(7)	Effect of treatment with the studied drugs for 2 weeks on HOMA-IR in male albino rats	119
(8)	Effect of treatment with the studied drugs for 2 weeks on serum triglycerides in male albino rats (mg/dl)	122
(9)	Effect of treatment with the studied drugs for 2 weeks on serum total cholesterol in male albino rats (mg/dl)	125
(10)	Effect of treatment with the studied drugs for 2 weeks on serum HDL-C in male albino rats (mg/dl)	128
(11)	Effect of treatment with the studied drugs for 2 weeks on serum LDL-C in male albino rats (mg/dl)	131
(12)	Effect of treatment with the studied drugs for 2 weeks on serum free fatty acids in male albino rats (mmol/L)	134
(13)	Effect of treatment with the studied drugs for 2 weeks on non-HDL-cholesterol in male albino rats (mg/dl)	137
(14)	Effect of treatment with the studied drugs for 2 weeks on triglycerides to HDL-cholesterol ratio in male albino rats	140
(15)	Effect of treatment with the studied drugs for 2 weeks on hepatic malondialdehyde in male albino rats (nmol/gm wet tissue)	143
(16)	Effect of treatment with the studied drugs for 2 weeks on hepatic reduced glutathione in male albino rats (μg/mg protein)	146

Table		Page
(17)	Effect of treatment with the studied drugs for 2 weeks on serum monocyte chemoattractant protein-1 in male albino rats (pg/ml)	**149**
(18)	Effect of treatment with the studied drugs for 2 weeks on serum C-reactive protein in male albino rats (mg/L)	**152**
(19)	Effect of treatment with the studied drugs for 2 weeks on serum nitric oxide in male albino rats (nmol/ml)	**155**

LIST OF FIGURES

Figure		Page
(1)	Model for the effects of adipocytes on pancreatic β-cell function/mass and insulin sensitivity in the pathogenesis of type 2 diabetes	10
(2)	Mitochondrial overproduction of superoxide activates the major pathways of hyperglycemic damage by inhibiting glyceraldehyde-3-phosphate dehydrogenase (GAPDH)	16
(3)	Development of type 2 diabetes	19
(4)	The cellular origins of reactive oxygen species, their targets, and antioxidant systems.	23
(5)	Schematic of the effects of chronic oxidative stress on the insulin signaling pathway	25
(6)	Structure of GSH (γ-glutamylcysteinyl glycine), where the N-terminal glutamate and cysteine are linked by the γ-carboxyl group of glutamate	29
(7)	Chemical structure of L-cysteine	32
(8)	The transsulfuration pathway in animals.	33
(9)	Sources and actions of cysteine and glutathione (GSH)	36
(10)	The role of serine kinase activation in oxidative stress-induced insulin resistance and the protective effect of some antioxidants by preserving the intracellular redox balance	37
(11)	Chemical structure of biguanides	41
(12)	Structure of human proinsulin and some commercially available insulin analogs.	57
(13)	Model of control of insulin release from the pancreatic β-cell by glucose and by sulfonylurea drugs	59
(14)	Schematic diagram of the insulin receptor heterodimer in the activated state.	60
(15)	Standard curve of insulin	73
(16)	Standard curve of Monocyte chemoattractant protein-1 (MCP-1)	82
(17)	Standard curve of nitric oxide	85
(18)	Standard curve of MDA	88
(19)	Standard curve of reduced glutathione	91
(20)	Standard curve of Protein	93
(21)	Effect of STZ-induced type 2 diabetes on fasting serum glucose in male albino rats	104

Figure		Page
(22)	Effect of STZ-induced type 2 diabetes on fasting serum insulin in male albino rats	104
(23)	Effect of STZ-induced type 2 diabetes on HOMA-IR in male albino rats	104
(24-a)	Effect of STZ-induced type 2 diabetes on serum triglycerides in male albino rats	106
(24-b)	Effect of STZ-induced type 2 diabetes on serum total cholesterol in male albino rats	106
(24-c)	Effect of STZ-induced type 2 diabetes on serum HDL-C in male albino rats	106
(24-d)	Effect of STZ-induced type 2 diabetes on serum LDL-C in male albino rats	106
(24-e)	Effect of STZ-induced type 2 diabetes on serum free fatty acids in male albino rats	107
(24-f)	Effect of STZ-induced type 2 diabetes on non- HDL-C in male albino rats	107
(24-g)	Effect of STZ-induced type 2 diabetes on TGs/HDL ratio in male albino rats	107
(25)	Effect of STZ-induced type 2 diabetes on hepatic malondialdehyde in male albino rats	109
(26)	Effect of STZ-induced type 2 diabetes on hepatic reduced glutathione in male albino rats	109
(27)	Effect of STZ-induced type 2 diabetes on serum monocyte chemoattractant protein-1 in male albino rats	111
(28)	Effect of STZ-induced type 2 diabetes on serum C-reactive protein in male albino rats	111
(29)	Effect of STZ-induced type 2 diabetes on serum nitric oxide in male albino rats	111
(30)	Effect of treatment with the studied drugs for 2 weeks on fasting serum glucose in male albino rats	114
(31)	Effect of treatment with the studied drugs for 2 weeks on fasting serum insulin in male albino rats	117
(32)	Effect of treatment with the studied drugs for 2 weeks on HOMA-IR in male albino rats	120
(33-a)	Effect of treatment with the studied drugs for 2 weeks on serum triglycerides in male albino rats	123
(33-b)	Effect of treatment with the studied drugs for 2 weeks on serum total cholesterol in male albino rats	126

Figure		Page
(33-c)	Effect of treatment with the studied drugs for 2 weeks on serum high density lipoprotein cholesterol in male albino rats	129
(33-d)	Effect of treatment with the studied drugs for 2 weeks on serum low density lipoprotein cholesterol in male albino rats	132
(33-e)	Effect of treatment with the studied drugs for 2 weeks on serum free fatty acids in male albino rats	135
(33-f)	Effect of treatment with the studied drugs for 2 weeks on non-HDL-cholesterol in male albino rats	138
(33-g)	Effect of treatment with the studied drugs for 2 weeks on triglycerides to HDL-cholesterol ratio in male albino rats	141
(34)	Effect of treatment with the studied drugs for 2 weeks on hepatic malondialdehyde in male albino rats	144
(35)	Effect of treatment with the studied drugs for 2 weeks on hepatic reduced glutathione in male albino rats	147
(36)	Effect of treatment with the studied drugs for 2 weeks on serum monocyte chemoattractant protein-1 in male albino rats	150
(37)	Effect of treatment with the studied drugs for 2 weeks on serum C-reactive protein in male albino rats	153
(38)	Effect of treatment with the studied drugs for 2 weeks on serum nitric oxide in male albino rats	156
(39)	Histopathological evaluation of pancreatic sections stained with hematoxylin and eosin (H&E) stain (X 10).	158
(40)	Comparison of mean percentage change in biochemical metabolic, oxidative stress and inflammatory parameters between untreated and treated (metformin, L-cysteine and their combination) experimentally induced type 2 diabetic adult male rats	159
(41)	Comparison of mean percentage change in lipid profile between untreated and treated (metformin, L-cysteine and their combination) experimentally induced type 2 diabetic adult male rats	160

LIST OF ABBREVIATIONS

8-OH-Guanine	:	8-hydroxy Guanine
ACC	:	Acetyl-CoA carboxylase
ACEI	:	Angiotensin converting enzyme inhibitors
ACOD	:	Acyl-CoA oxidase
Acyl CS	:	Acyl CoA synthetase
ADP	:	Adenosine diphosphate
AGEs	:	Advanced glycation endproducts
AIDS	:	Acquired immunodeficiency syndrome
Akt	:	Apoptosis serine/therionine kinase
AMP	:	Adenosine monophosphate
AMPK	:	Adenosine monophosphate-activated protein kinase
ARB	:	Angiotensin receptor blocker
ATP	:	Adenosine triphosphate
ATPase	:	Adenosinine triphosphatase enzyme
BH$_4$	:	Tetrahydrobiopterin cofactor
Ca^{2+}	:	Calcium ion
CAT	:	Catalase
Ccl2	:	Chemokine ligand 2
CCl$_4$	:	Carbon tetrachloride
Ccr2	:	Cognate receptor chemokine receptor 2
CD4	:	Cluster of differentiation 4
cNOS	:	Constitutive nitric oxide synthase
CoA	:	Coenzyme A
CoQ$_{10}$	:	Coenzyme Q$_{10}$
CRP	:	C-reactive protein
Cu	:	Cupper
Cu/Zn SOD	:	Cupper zinc superoxide dismutase
DAG	:	Diacylglycerol
DHAP	:	dihydroxyacetone phosphate
DM	:	Diabetes mellitus

DNA	:	Deoxyribonucleic acid
DPP-4	:	Dipeptidyl peptidase-4
DTNB	:	5,5'-Dithiobis-2-nitrobenzoic acid
ECS	:	Endocannabinoid system
EDTA	:	Disodium salt of ethylene diamine tetraacetic acid
ELISA	:	Enzyme linked immunosorbent assay
eNOS	:	Endothelial nitric oxide synthase
ESRF	:	End stage renal failure
ETC	:	Electron transport chain
FADH$_2$	:	Reduced flavin-adenine dinucleotide
FAS	:	Fatty acid synthase
FBPase	:	Fructose 1,6-bisphosphatase
FDA	:	Food and drug administration
Fe	:	Iron
FFAs	:	Free fatty acids
FSG	:	Fasting serum glucose
FSI	:	Fasting serum insulin
GADA	:	Glutamic acid decarboxylase autoantibodies
GAPDH	:	Glyceraldehyde-3-phosphate dehydrogenase
GDM	:	Gestational diabetes mellitus
GFAT	:	Glutamine:fructose-6-phosphate amidotransferase
GIP	:	Gastric inhibitory polypeptide
Gln	:	Glutamine
GLP-1	:	Glucagon-like peptide-1
Glu	:	Glutamate
GLUT1	:	Glucose transporter-1
GLUT2	:	Glucose transporter-2
GLUT3	:	Glucose transporter-3
GLUT4	:	Glucose transporter-4
GPx	:	Glutathione peroxidase
GSH	:	Reduced glutathione
GSSG	:	Oxidized glutathione
GST	:	Glutathione transferase

H_2O	:	Water molecule
H_2O_2	:	Hydrogen peroxide
HBA_{1C}	:	Glycated Hemoglobin A_{1C}
HCl	:	Hydrochloric acid
HDL-C	:	High density lipoprotein cholesterol
HFD	:	High fat diet
HIV-1	:	Human immunodeficiency virus-1
HLA	:	Human leukocyte antigen
HMG-CoA	:	3-hydroxy-3-methyl-glutaryl-Coenzyme A
HNF-1α	:	Hepatic nuclear factor-1 α
HNF-4α	:	Hepatic nuclear factor-4 α
HNO_2	:	Nitrous oxide
HOCL	:	Hypochlorous acid
HOMA-IR	:	Homeostasis model assessment of insulin resistance
$HRO_2^{\bullet}$	:	Hydroperoxyl
HRP	:	Horseradish peroxidase enzyme
IAAs	:	Insulin autoantibodies
ICAM-1	:	Intercellular adhesion molecule-1
ICAs	:	Islet-cell autoantibodies
IDL	:	Intermediate density lipoprotein
IGT	:	Impaired glucose tolerance
IKKβ	:	Inhibitor of nuclear factor-κB kinase beta
IL-1	:	Interleukin-1
IL-10	:	Interleukin-10
IL-2	:	Interleukin-2
IL-6	:	Interleukin-6
IL-8	:	Interleukin-8
iNOS	:	Inducible nitric oxide synthase
IPF-1	:	Insulin promoter factor-1
IR	:	Insulin resistance
IRS-1	:	Insulin receptor substrate-1
K^+/Na^+ tartarate	:	Potassium sodium tartarate

K⁺ATP channels	:	Potassium channels adenosine triphosphate
KCl	:	Potassium chloride
LADA	:	Latent autoimmune diabetes in adults
LDL-C	:	Low density lipoprotein cholesterol
LPL	:	Lipoprotein lipase
LSD	:	Least significant difference
MAOIs	:	Monoamine oxidase inhibitors
MCP-1	:	Monocyte chemoattractant protein-1
MDA	:	Malondialdehyde
microRNA	:	micro-ribonucleic acid
Mn-SOD	:	Manganese superoxide dismutase
MODY	:	Maturity onset diabetes of the young
mRNA	:	Messenger ribonucleic acid
NAC	:	N-acetyl cysteine
NAD⁺	:	Oxidized nicotinamide-adenine dinucleotide
NADH	:	Reduced nicotinanide adenine dinucleotide
NADP	:	Oxidized Nicotinamide adenine dinucleotide phosphate
NADPH	:	Reduced Nicotinamide adenine dinucleotide phosphate
NaOH	:	Sodium hydroxide
NED	:	N-(1-naphthyl) ethylenediamine
NEFA	:	Non-esterified fatty acids
NF-κB	:	Nuclear factor kappa B
nNOS	:	Neural nitric oxide synthase
NO	:	Nitric oxide
NO_2^-	:	Nitrite
$NO_2^{\bullet-}$	:	Nitrogen dioxide
NO_3^-	:	Nitrate
Non-HDL-C	:	Non-high density lipoprotein cholesterol
NPH	:	Neutral protamine
NSAIDs	:	Non steroidal anti-inflammatory drugs
O₂	:	Oxygen molecule

$O_2^{\bullet-}$	:	Superoxide radical
OCT1	:	Organic cation transporter-1
$OH^{\bullet}$	:	Hydroxyl radical
$ONOO^-$	:	Peroxynitre
P	:	Phosphate
PAI-1	:	Plasminogen-activator inhibitor -1
PCOS	:	Polycystic ovarian syndrome
PDX-1	:	Pancreas duodenum homeobox-1
PEPCK	:	Phosphenolpyruvate carboxykinase
PI3K	:	Phosphatidylinositol 3-kinase
PKC	:	Protein kinase C
PPAR-α	:	Peroxisome proliferator-activated receptor alpha
PPAR-γ	:	Peroxisome proliferator-activated receptor gamma
Prx	:	Peroxiredoxin
PUFAs	:	Polyunsaturated fatty acids
RAGE	:	Receptor for advanced glycation endproducts
rDNA	:	Recombinant deoxyribonucleic acid
RNS	:	Reactive nitrogen species
$RO_2^{\bullet}$	:	Proxyl radical
RONOO	:	Alkyl peroxynitrates
ROS	:	Reactive oxygen species
rpm	:	Rotation per minute
SDS	:	Sodecyl sulphate
SGLT2	:	Sodium-glucose cotransporter-2
SH	:	Thiol or sulfhydryl group
SOD	:	Superoxide dismutase
SREBP	:	Sterol regulatory element-binding protein
STZ	:	Streptozotocin
SUR1	:	Sulfonylurea receptor 1
SUs	:	Sulfonylureas
T1DM	:	Type 1 diabetes mellitus
T2DM	:	Type 2 diabetes mellitus

TBA	:	Thiobarbituric acid
TBARS	:	Thiobarbituric acid reactive substances
TBHB	:	2,4,4-tribromo-3-hydroxy-benzoic acid
TC	:	Total cholesterol
TCA	:	Trichloroacetic acid
TGs	:	Triglycerides
TMB	:	3,3',5,5' tetramethylbenzidine
TMP	:	1,1, 3,3-tetramethoxypropane
TNB	:	5-thionitrobenzoic acid
TNF-α	:	Tumor necrosis factor-α
Trx	:	Thioredoxin
TxA2	:	Thromboxane A2
Tyr	:	Tyrosine
TZDs	:	Thiazolidinediones
UDP-GlcNac	:	Uridine diphospho-N-acetylglucosamine
VCAM-1	:	Vascular cell adhesion molecule-1
VEGF	:	Vascular endothelial growth factor
VLDL	:	Very low density lipoproteins
WHO	:	World Health Organization
ZDF	:	Zucker diabetic fatty
Zn	:	Zinc

BACKGROUND OF THE STUDY

Diabetes mellitus (DM) is a chronic multisystem disorder with biochemical consequences and serious complications that affect many organs. There are complex interactions between genetic, epigenetic, environmental and behavioural factors that contribute to the development of diabetes. Non-pharmacological and pharmacological interventions have been used for diabetic management. Over the past few years, research has started to focus on the use of novel adjuvant drugs as antioxidants and anti-inflammatory drugs for better management, as it was revealed that both oxidative stress and inflammation play a critical role in the disease pathogenesis.

Metformin is a widely used oral antidiabetic agent for the management of type 2 diabetes. Its primary mode of action appears to be through improvement of insulin sensitivity and suppression of hepatic gluconeogenesis and glycogenolysis. Moreover, it affects glucose transport system, increases glucose utilization and delays its absorption from the intestine. It also shows beneficial effects on diabetes, as weight reduction and improvements in lipid profile, inflammation and endothelial function.

L-cysteine is a semi-essential sulfur containing amino acid. One important function of L-cysteine is that it is a precursor of glutathione, which is pivotal for the detoxification of cellular oxidative stress. Dietary intake of cysteine-rich proteins lowers the oxidative stress and insulin resistance. It improves glycemic control, shows an anti-inflammatory effect and implies a protective effect on pancreatic β-cells.

Taking the above mentioned data in consideration, it seems that combined therapy of metformin and an antioxidant like L-cysteine may be of value in treatment of the diabetic state and amelioration of the oxidative stress and inflammation associated with diabetes mellitus.

INTRODUCTION

Diabetes mellitus is the most common endocrine metabolic disorder, affecting about 170 million people worldwide [1]. It represents a group of diseases with complex heterogeneous etiology, characterized by chronic hyperglycemia with carbohydrate, fat and protein metabolic abnormalities[2], which are due to insulin deficiency and/or insulin resistance [3]. These abnormalities result in the impairment of uptake and storage of glucose and reduced glucose utilization for energy purposes. Defects in glucose metabolizing machinery and consistent efforts of the physiological system to correct the imbalance in glucose metabolism place an over-exertion on the endocrine system. Continuing deterioration of endocrine control exacerbates the metabolic disturbances and leads primarily to hyperglycemia[4], then proceeds to the development of long-term complications, such as microangiopathy; nephropathy, neuropathy and retinopathy. The basis of these complications is a subject of great debate and research. Hyperglycemia and metabolic derangement are accused as the main causes of these long-standing changes in various organs. Hyperglycemia may also lead to increased generation of free radicals and reduced antioxidant defense system [3].

Epidemiology of diabetes mellitus

Diabetes mellitus is a common growing disease, which is considered epidemic by WHO. Its incidence in adults and adolescents have been alarmingly rising in developed countries with estimate for an increase of 60% in the adult population above 30 years of age in 2025, with a higher prevalence in the 45 to 64 years-old adults [5]. These increases are expected because of population ageing and urbanization. According to the WHO, undiagnosed diabetes in Egypt will be about 8.8 million by the year 2025[6].

Diabetes mellitus classification

The current classification includes four main categories [7]:

I- Type 1 diabetes, either type 1A (immune-mediated, e.g. latent autoimmune diabetes in adults [LADA]) or type 1 B (idiopathic)

II- Type 2 diabetes

III- Other specific types

1. Genetic defects of β-cell function (maturity onset diabetes of the young [MODY]). These defects may be in genes of hepatic nuclear factor (HNF-1α or HNF-4α) or insulin promoter factor-1 (IPF-1).
2. Genetic defects in insulin action (Type A insulin resistance, lipoatrophic diabetes).
3. Diseases of the exocrine pancreas (pancreatitis, neoplasia, cystic fibrosis, hemochromatosis).
4. Endocrinopathies (acromegaly, Cushing's syndrome, glucagonoma, pheochromocytoma, hyperthyroidism).
5. Drug or chemical induced (vacor, streptozotocin, alloxan, glucocorticoids, thyroid hormone, diazoxide, thiazide diuretics, minoxidil, oral contraceptives, L-dopa).
6. Infections (congenital rubella, cytomegalovirus).
7. Uncommon forms of immune-mediated diabetes ("Stiff-man" syndrome, anti-insulin receptor antibodies).
8. Other genetic syndromes sometimes associated with diabetes (Down syndrome, Klinefelter syndrome, Turner syndrome).

IV-Gestational diabetes mellitus

Gestational diabetes mellitus (GDM) is defined as any abnormal carbohydrate intolerance that begins or is first recognized during pregnancy[8]. It is associated with an increased risk of perinatal mortality and congenital abnormalities, which is further increased by impaired glycemic control [9]. It occurs in approximately 7% of all pregnancies and if occurred once, it is likely to occur in subsequent pregnancies. Up to 70% of women with GDM have a potential risk of developing type 2 diabetes mellitus. The risk factors for developing gestational diabetes are similar to those for type 2 diabetes, including family history, age, obesity and ethnicity [10]. It is known that pregnancy is a diabetogenic state, characterized by impaired insulin sensitivity, particularly in the second and third trimester. This is due to changes in some hormones such as human placental lactogen, progesterone, prolactin and cortisol that antagonize the effects of insulin and decrease phosphorylation of insulin receptor substrate-1 (IRS-1), triggering a state of insulin resistance. Logically, the pancreas should compensate for this demand by increasing insulin secretion. However in GDM, there is deterioration of beta cell function, particularly the first phase insulin secretion [8].

An intermediate group of individuals with impaired fasting glucose and/or impaired glucose tolerance was classified as "pre-diabetics". Their progression to diabetes is common, particularly when non-pharmacological interventions, such as lifestyle changes are not provided [7].

I-Type 1 diabetes mellitus

Type 1 diabetes mellitus (T1DM) is an organ-specific progressive cellular-mediated autoimmune disease characterized by a defect in insulin production, as a result of selective and massive destruction of islet β-cells (80–90%). It accounts for only about 5–10% of all cases of diabetes; however, its incidence continues to increase worldwide. The progression of the autoimmune process is generally slow and may take several years before the onset of the clinical diabetes [11]. Markers of the immune β-cell destruction, including circulating insulin autoantibodies (IAAs), islet-cell autoantibodies (ICAs) and glutamic acid decarboxylase autoantibodies (GADA), are present in 90% of patients at the time of diagnosis [7].

Two forms are identified:

- Type 1A DM, which results from a cell-mediated autoimmune attack on β-cells and has a strong genetic component, inherited through the human leukocyte antigen (HLA) complex, mainly HLA-DR3 and HLA-DR4 [12], but the factors that trigger onset of clinical disease remain largely unknown.

- Type 1B DM (idiopathic) is a far less frequent form, has no known cause, and occurs mostly in individuals of Asian or African descent[7]. This form of diabetes lacks evidence for β-cell autoimmunity and is not HLA associated. While the disease is often manifested by severe insulinopenia and/or ketoacidosis, β-cell function often recovers, rendering almost normal glucose levels [13].

Starting generally at a young age, T1DM is also referred to as 'juvenile diabetes'. Indeed, it affects children and young adults in particular and generally occurs before the age of 40, with incidence peaks at 2, 4-6 and 10-14 years [11]. However, it can also occur at any age, even as late as in the eighth and ninth decades of life. The slow rate of β-cell destruction in adults may mask the presentation, making it difficult to distinguish from type 2 diabetes. This type of diabetes is known as "Latent Autoimmune Diabetes in Adults" [13].

Patients with type 1 diabetes are severely insulin deficient and are dependent on insulin replacement therapy for their survival [13].

II-Type 2 diabetes mellitus

Type 2 diabetes mellitus (T2DM) is a complex metabolic disorder of polygenic nature, that is characterized by defects in both insulin action and insulin secretion [14]. T2DM affects nowadays more than 150 million people worldwide and is projected to increase to 439 million worldwide in 2030[15]. By the end of the 20th century, its incidence has increased dramatically in children and adolescents, as a result of the rise in childhood obesity and is now continuing to rise, changing the demographics of the disease in this group [16].

Genetic, epigenetic and environmental factors have been implicated in type 2 diabetes mellitus pathogenesis with increasing evidences that epigenetic factors play a key role in the complex interplay between them[17]. Epigenetic mechanisms are commonly associated to gene silencing and transcriptional regulation of genes [18]. The epigenetic control of gene expression is based on modulation of chromatin structure and accessibility to transcription factors, which is achieved by multiple mechanisms. These mechanisms involve methylation–demethylation of cytidine–guanosine sequences in the promoter regions, acetylation–deacetylation of lysine residues of core histones in the nucleosome and presence of microRNA molecules, which bind to their complementary sequences in the 3′ end of mRNA and reduce the rate of protein synthesis[19]. Actions of major pathological mediators of diabetes and its complications such as hyperglycemia, oxidative stress and inflammation can lead to the dysregulation of these epigenetic mechanisms [17].

Insulin resistance in peripheral tissues, such as muscle and fat, is often the earliest recognizable feature of T2DM, results in a compensatory hyperinsulinemia that promotes further weight gain. This occurs until the β-cells can no longer compensate for the increased insulin resistance, then β-cell failure and hyperglycemia ensue [20]. It is also associated with co-morbidities, such as hypertension, hyperlipidemia and cardiovascular diseases, which taken together comprise the 'Metabolic Syndrome' [20].

Similar to adults, obesity in children appears to be a major risk factor for type 2 diabetes [21]. Many studies show a strong family history among affected youth, with 45-80% having at least one parent with diabetes and 74-100% having a first- or second-degree relative with type 2 diabetes [22]. Until now, type 2 diabetes was typically regarded as a disease of the middle-aged and elderly. While it is still true that this age group maintains a higher risk than the younger adults do, evidence is accumulating that onset in children and adolescents is increasingly common. Onset of diabetes in childhood or adolescence, around the time of puberty, heralds many years of disease and increases the risk of occurrence of the full range of both micro- and macrovascular complications [23].

Although a mother could transmit genetic susceptibility to her offspring, it is more likely that maternal diabetes increases the risk of diabetes in children by altering the intrauterine environment, which can impair the normal β-cell development and function as well as the insulin sensitivity of skeletal muscle [24]. Moreover, malnutrition during fetal or early life and low birth weight appear to be associated with an increased risk of adulthood insulin resistance, glucose intolerance, T2DM, dyslipidemia and hypertension [25].

Normal glucose homeostasis

Maintenance of serum glucose concentrations within a normal physiological range (fasting blood glucose level 70-110 mg/dl), is primarily accomplished by two pancreatic hormones; insulin, secreted by the β-cells and glucagon, secreted by α-cells [26]. Derangements of glucagon or insulin regulation can result in hyperglycemia or hypoglycemia, respectively.

In the postabsorptive state, the majority of total body glucose disposal takes place in insulin-independent tissues [27]. Approximately 50% of all glucose utilization occurs in the brain and 25% of glucose uptake occurs in the splanchnic area (liver and the gastrointestinal tissue). The remaining 25% of glucose metabolism takes place in insulin-dependent tissues, primarily muscle with only a small amount being metabolized by adipocytes [28]. Approximately 85% of endogenous glucose production is derived from the liver and the remaining amount is produced by the kidney. Glycogenolysis and gluconeogenesis contribute equally to the basal rate of hepatic glucose production [27].

In the postprandial state, the maintenance of whole-body glucose homeostasis is dependent upon a normal insulin secretory response and normal tissue sensitivity to the effects of hyperinsulinemia and hyperglycemia to augment glucose disposal. This occurs by three tightly coupled mechanisms: (i) suppression of endogenous glucose production and increase glycogen synthesis; (ii) stimulation of glucose uptake by the splanchnic tissues; and (iii) stimulation of glucose uptake by peripheral tissues, primarily muscle [27].

The route of glucose administration also plays an important role in the overall glucose homeostasis. Oral glucose ingestion has a potentiating effect on insulin secretion that the insulin concentrations in the circulation increase very rapidly (by at least two to threefold) after oral glucose, when compared to a similar intravenous bolus of glucose. This potentiating effect of oral glucose administration is known as "the incretin effect" and is related to the release of glucagon-like peptide-1 (GLP-1) and glucose-dependent insulinotropic polypeptide (also called gastric inhibitory polypeptide) (GIP) from the gastrointestinal tissues [29].

Glucose homeostasis in type 2 diabetes mellitus

Type 2 diabetic individuals are characterized by defects in insulin secretion; insulin resistance involving muscle, liver and the adipocytes; and abnormalities in splanchnic glucose uptake [28].

Insulin secretion in insulin resistant, non-diabetic individuals is increased in proportion to the severity of the insulin resistance and glucose tolerance remains normal. Thus, their pancreas is able to "read" the severity of insulin resistance and adjust its secretion of insulin. However, the progression to type 2 diabetes with mild fasting hyperglycemia (120-140 mg/dl) is heralded by an inability of the β-cell to maintain its previously high rate of insulin secretion in response to a glucose challenge, without any further or only minimal deterioration in tissue sensitivity to insulin [27].

The relationship between the fasting plasma glucose concentration and the fasting plasma insulin concentration resembles an inverted U or horseshoe. As the fasting plasma glucose concentration rises from 80 to 140 mg/dl, the fasting plasma insulin concentration increases progressively, peaking at a value that is 2-2.5 folds greater than in normal weight, non-diabetic, age-matched controls. The progressive rise in fasting plasma insulin level can be viewed as an adaptive response of the pancreas to offset the progressive deterioration in glucose homeostasis. However, when the fasting plasma glucose concentration exceeds 140 mg/dl, the beta cell is unable to maintain its elevated rate of insulin secretion and the fasting insulin concentration declines precipitously. This decrease in fasting insulin level has important physiologic implications, since at this point; hepatic glucose production begins to rise, which is correlated with the severity of fasting and postprandial hyperglycemia [27].

Moreover, the largest part of the impairment in insulin-mediated glucose uptake is accounted for a defect in muscle glucose disposal. Thus in the basal state, the liver represents a major site of insulin resistance [30]; however in the postprandial state, both decreased muscle glucose uptake and impaired suppression of hepatic glucose production contribute to the insulin resistance, together with defect in insulin secretion, are the causes of postprandial hyperglycemia. It should be noted that brain glucose uptake occurs at the same rate during absorptive and postabsorptive periods and is not altered in type 2 diabetes [28].

Pathophysiology of type 2 diabetes mellitus

Insulin resistance:

Insulin resistance (IR) is the impaired sensitivity and attenuated response to insulin in its main target organs, adipose tissue, liver, and muscle, leading to compensatory hyperinsulinemia [31].

In adipose tissue, insulin decreases lipolysis, thereby reducing FFAs efflux from the adipocytes. However, intra-abdominal fat is metabolically distinct from subcutaneous fat, as it is more lipolytically active and less sensitive to the antilipolytic effects of insulin. In liver, insulin inhibits gluconeogenesis by reducing key enzyme activities. While in skeletal muscle, insulin predominantly induces glucose uptake by stimulating the translocation of the GLUT4 glucose transporter to the plasma membrane and promotes glycogen synthesis [32].

Insulin resistance leads to increased lipolysis of the stored triacylglycerol molecules with subsequent increase circulating FFAs concentrations and ectopic fat accumulation. This results in increases in the flux of FFAs from fat to liver and periphery. Excess delivery of FFAs stimulates liver glucose and triglycerides production [33], impedes insulin mediated glucose uptake and decreases glycogen synthesis in skeletal muscle [34], as well as impairs vascular reactivity and induces inflammation[35]. This is shown in Figure (1).

At the molecular level, impaired insulin signaling results from reduced receptor expression or mutations or post-translational modifications of the insulin receptor itself or any of its downstream effector molecules. These reduce tyrosine-specific protein kinase activity or its ability to phosphorylate substrate proteins (IRS) [36] resulting in phosphatidylinositol-3-kinase (PI3K)/Akt pathway impairment [37].

To date, several methods for evaluating insulin resistance in humans have been reported such as fasting serum insulin levels, homeostasis model assessment of insulin resistance (HOMA-IR) and insulin tolerance test [38]. Because abnormalities in insulin action are poorly detected by a single determination of either glucose or insulin levels, the insulin resistance is commonly evaluated by HOMA-IR, which is likely to be the most simple and repeatable index [38, 39].

Glucotoxicity:

Insulin resistance results in chronic fasting and postprandial hyperglycemia. Chronic hyperglycemia may deplete insulin secretory granules from β-cells, leaving less insulin ready for release in response to a new glucose stimulus [40]. This has led to the concept of glucose toxicity, which implies the development of irreversible damage to cellular components of insulin production over time. Hyperglycemia stimulates the production of large amounts of reactive oxygen species (ROS) in β-cells. Due to ROS interference, loss of pancreas duodenum homeobox-1 (PDX-1) has been proposed as an important mechanism leading to β-cell dysfunction. PDX-1 is a necessary transcription factor for insulin gene expression and glucose-induced insulin secretion, besides being a critical regulator of β-cell survival. Additionally, ROS are known to enhance NF-κB activity, which potentially induces β-cell apoptosis [41].

Lipotoxicity:

Chronically elevated free fatty acids (FFAs) level results from the resistance to the antipolytic effect of insulin. It is known that FFAs acutely stimulate insulin secretion, but chronically impair insulin secretion, induce further hepatic and muscle insulin resistance, stimulate gluconeogenesis and cause a decrease β-cell function and mass, an effect referred to as β-cell lipotoxicity [42].

In the presence of glucose, fatty acid oxidation in β-cells is inhibited and accumulation of long-chain acyl coenzyme A occurs. This mechanism has been proposed to be an integral part of the normal insulin secretory process. However, its excessive accumulation can diminish the insulin secretory process by opening β-cell potassium channels. Another mechanism might involve apoptosis of β-cells, possibly via generation of nitric oxide through inducible nitric oxide synthase (iNOS) activation which results in great production of toxic peroxynitrite (ONOO⁻) [43].

Thus, glucolipotoxicity may play an important role in the pathogenesis of hyperglycemia and dyslipidemia associated with type 2 diabetes [44].

Dyslipidemia:

Diabetic dyslipidemia is typically defined by its characteristic lipid 'triad' profile, known as atherogenic dyslipidemia, which is usually an increase in plasma triglycerides, a decrease in high-density lipoprotein cholesterol and a concomitant increase in small dense oxidized low-density lipoproteins [45, 46]. These lipid abnormalities may be a more important risk factor for atherosclerosis and cardiovascular diseases than hyperglycemia [46].

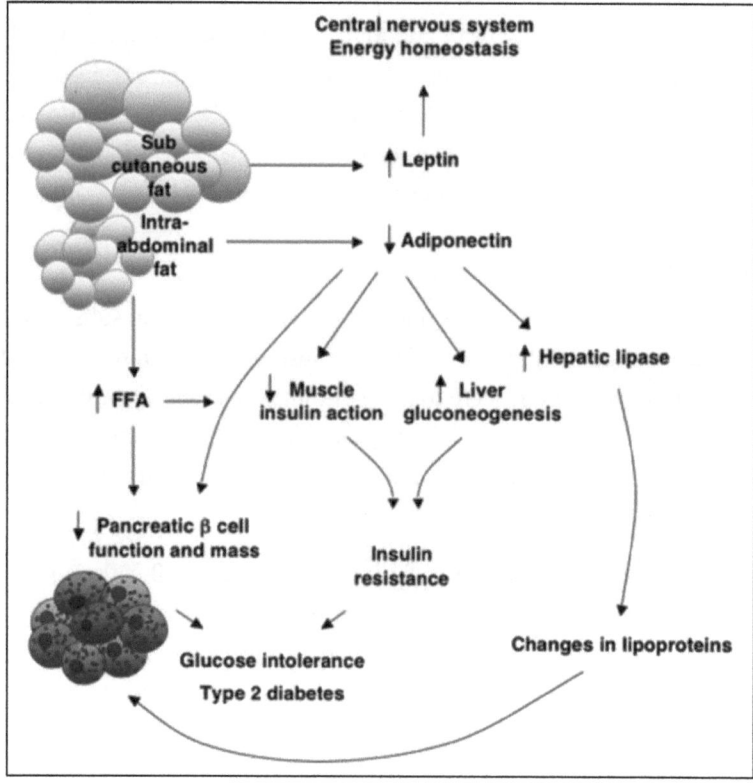

Figure (1): Model for the effects of adipocytes on pancreatic β-cell function/mass and insulin sensitivity in the pathogenesis of type 2 diabetes [47].

In diabetic patients, there is typically a preponderance of smaller, denser, oxidized LDL particles, which may increase atherogenicity and cardiovascular risk, even if the absolute concentration of LDL cholesterol is not elevated [45].

Non-HDL cholesterol (non-HDL-C) is a new measure that reflects the combined lipid profile change. It encompasses all cholesterol present in the potentially atherogenic lipoprotein particles (VLDL, remnants, IDL and LDL). Non-HDL-C has been shown to correlate with coronary artery disease severity and progression, as well as predicts cardiovascular morbidity and mortality in patients with diabetes [48].

Another simple tool, Triglycerides to HDL-cholesterol ratio (TGs: HDL-C) has been proposed as an atherogenic index, that has proven to be a highly significant predictor of myocardial infarction, even stronger than total cholesterol to HDL-C ratio and LDL-C to HDL-C ratio [49]. Moreover, a significant negative relationship between TGs: HDL-C ratio and insulin sensitivity was observed. Thus a TGs: HDL-C ratio ≥ 3.5 provides a simple mean of identifying insulin resistant, dyslipidemic patients who are at increased risk of cardiovascular diseases[50].

The precise pathogenesis of diabetic dyslipidemia is not fully known; nevertheless, a large body of evidence suggests that insulin resistance has a central role in the development of this condition as a result of the increased influx of free fatty acids from insulin-resistant fat cells into the liver, in the presence of adequate glycogen stores[51].

Diabetic complications and their pathogenesis

Hyperosmolar hyperglycemic non-ketotic state

It is one of the major acute complications, which is a life-threatening condition, commonly occurs in elderly patients with type 2 diabetes. There is almost always a precipitating factor which include; the use of some drugs, acute situations and chronic diseases. Abnormal thirst sensation and limited access to water also facilitate development of this syndrome. It is associated with four major clinical features, which are severe hyperglycemia (blood glucose more than 600 mg/dl), absent or slight ketosis, plasma hyperosmolarity and profound dehydration. Treatment of this state should be started immediately with the determination and correction of the precipitating event and lifesaving measures, while the other clinical manifestations should be corrected with the use of appropriate fluids and insulin [52].

However, chronic complications can be divided into microvascular; affecting eyes, kidneys and nerves and macrovascular; affecting the coronary, cerebral and peripheral vascular systems [53].

Microvascular complications

In fact, microvascular complications can begin in developing at least 7 years before the clinical diagnosis of type 2 diabetes. Conversely; type 1 patients may not develop signs of microvascular complications until 10 years after diagnosis of diabetes [54].

Nephropathy: Diabetic nephropathy is a frequent complication of type 1 and type 2 diabetes mellitus, characterized by excessive urinary albumin excretion, hypertension and progressive renal insufficiency. The natural history of diabetic nephropathy has 5 stages; which include hyperfiltration with normal renal function; histological changes without clinically evident disease; incipient diabetic nephropathy or microalbuminuria; overt diabetic nephropathy (macroalbuminuria and reduced renal function); and renal failure requiring dialysis (end stage renal disease) [55].

Neuropathy: Diabetic peripheral neuropathy is one of the most prevalent and complicated conditions to manage among diabetic patients. Diabetes is the major contributing reason for non-traumatic lower extremity amputations (more than 60% of cases). Ischemia occurs because of compromised vasculature that fails to deliver oxygen and nutrients to nerve fibers. This results in damage to myelin sheath covering and insulating nerve. The most common form involves the somatic nervous system; however, the autonomic nervous system may be affected in some patients. Sensorimotor neuropathy is characterized by symptoms; such as burning, tingling sensations and allodynia. Autonomic neuropathy can cause gastroparesis, sexual dysfunction and bladder incontinence [54].

Retinopathy: Diabetic retinopathy is the most frequent cause of new cases of blindness among adults aged 20-74 years [56]. Non-proliferative retinopathy produces blood vessel changes within the retina, which include weakened blood vessel walls, leakage of fluids and loss of circulation. It generally does not interfere with vision [54]. However, if left untreated, it can progress to proliferative retinopathy, that is very serious and severe. It occurs when new blood vessels branch out or proliferate in and around the retina [56]. It can cause bleeding into the fluid-filled center of the eye or swelling of the retina, leading to blindness. The duration of diabetes and the degree of hyperglycemia are probably the strongest predictors for development and progression of retinopathy [54].

Macrovascular complications

The hallmark of diabetic macrovascular disease is the accelerated atherosclerosis; involving the aorta and the large and medium-sized arteries, which is a leading cause of morbidity and mortality in diabetes [54]. Accelerated atherosclerosis caused by accumulation of lipoproteins within the vessel wall, resulting in the increased formation of fibrous plaques [53]. Hyperglycemia also affects endothelial function, resulting in increased permeability, altered release of vasoactive substances, increased production of procoagulation proteins and decreased production of fibrinolytic factors [53]. All these changes result in atherosclerotic heart disease, myocardial infarction and sudden death; peripheral vascular disease and cerebrovascular disease, including cerebral hemorrhage, infarction and stroke.

Hyperglycemia causes tissue damage through four major mechanisms. Several evidences indicate that all these mechanisms are activated by a single upstream event, which is the mitochondrial overproduction of reactive oxygen species [57], Figure (2).

Increased polyol pathway flux

The polyol pathway is based on a family of aldo-keto reductase enzymes, which can use as substrates a wide variety of carbonyl compounds and reduce them by NADPH to their respective sugar alcohols (polyols). Glucose is converted to sorbitol by the enzyme aldose reductase, which is then oxidized to fructose by the enzyme sorbitol dehydrogenase, using NAD^+ as a cofactor. Aldose reductase is found in tissues such as nerve, retina, lens, glomerulus and vascular cells. In many of these tissues, glucose uptake is mediated by insulin-independent GLUTs; intracellular glucose concentrations, therefore, rise in parallel with hyperglycemia [57].

Several mechanisms include sorbitol-induced osmotic stress, increased cytosolic $NADH/NAD^+$ and decreased cytosolic NADPH have been proposed to explain tissue damage resulted from this pathway [58]. The most cited is an increase in redox stress, caused by the consumption of NADPH, a cofactor required to regenerate reduced glutathione (GSH), which is an important scavenger of ROS. This could induce or exacerbate intracellular oxidative stress [57].

Increased intracellular advanced glycation endproducts (AGEs) formation and increased expression of the receptor for AGEs (RAGE)

AGEs are formed by the non-enzymatic reaction of glucose and other glycating compounds derived both from glucose and fatty acids with proteins [59]. Intracellular production of AGE precursors can damage cells by altering protein functions and binding of plasma proteins modified by AGE precursors to RAGE on cells such as macrophages and vascular endothelial cells. RAGE binding induces the production of ROS, which in turn activates the pleiotropic transcription factor nuclear factor (NF-κB), causing multiple pathological changes in gene expression [60]. These effects induce procoagulatory changes and increase the adhesion of inflammatory cells to the endothelium. In addition, this binding appears to mediate, in part, the increased vascular permeability induced by diabetes, probably through the induction of VEGF [57].

Increased protein kinase C (PKC) activation

PKC activation results primarily from enhanced de-novo synthesis of diacylglycerol (DAG) from glucose via triose phosphate. Evidence suggests that the enhanced activity of PKC isoforms could also result from the interaction between AGEs and their cell-surface receptors [57]. PKC activation implicated in many processes; such as increased vascular permeability, angiogenesis, blood flow abnormalities, capillary and vascular occlusion, which are involved in the pathology of diabetic complications [58].

Increased hexosamine pathway flux

Hyperglycemia and elevated free fatty acids also appear to contribute to the pathogenesis of diabetic complications by increasing the flux of glucose and fructose-6-phophate into the hexosamine pathway, leading to increases in the transcription of some key genes and alteration in protein functions such as eNOS inhibition [57].

Mitochondrial superoxide overproduction

It has now been established that all of the different pathogenic mechanisms described above stem from a single hyperglycemia-induced process, namely overproduction of superoxide by the mitochondrial electron-transport chain that can damage cells in numerous ways. It is hypothesized that excess ROS inhibits GAPDH (glyceraldehyde-3-phosphate dehydrogenase), a glycolytic key enzyme promoting shunting of upstream glucose metabolites into the aforementioned pathways [57]. This overproduction of ROS can be prevented by manganese superoxide dismutase [61].

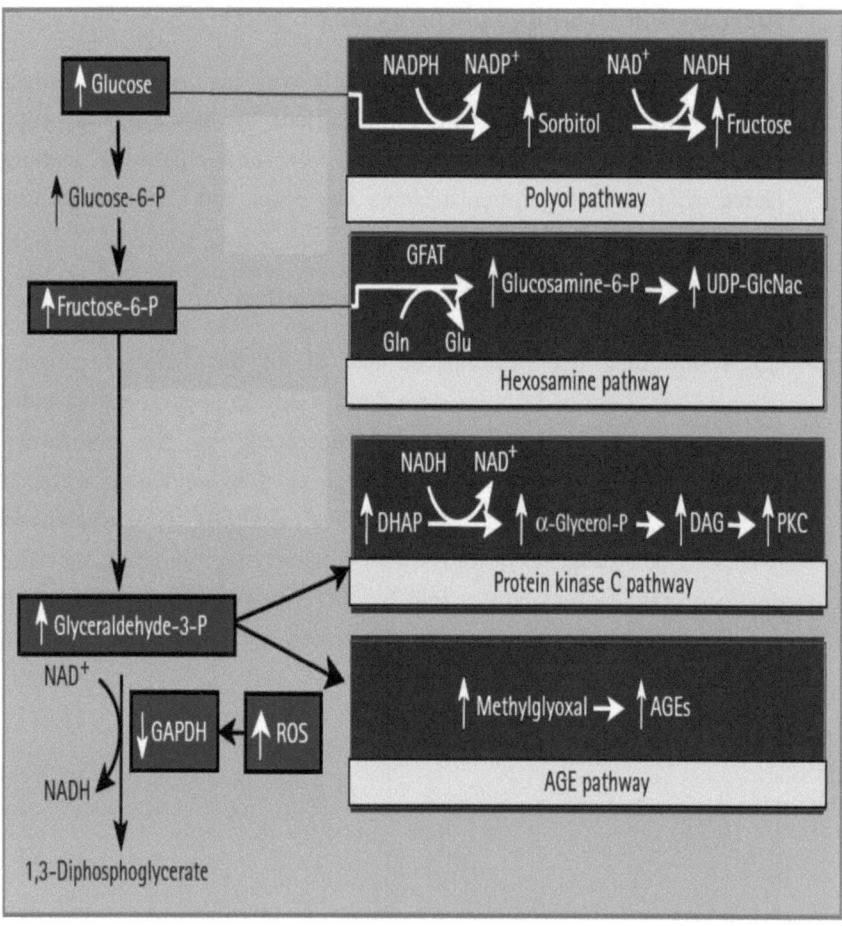

Figure (2): Mitochondrial overproduction of superoxide activates the major pathways of hyperglycemic damage by inhibiting glyceraldehyde-3-phosphate dehydrogenase (GAPDH) [62].

Obesity, inflammation and insulin resistance

Although genetic predisposition to insulin resistance exists, it is widely accepted that the increasingly sedentary lifestyle; such as consumption of a high caloric diet and lack of exercise, have increased the global prevalence of not only insulin resistance and diabetes, but also of obesity [63]. Between 60% and 90% of cases of type 2 diabetes now appear to be related to obesity [64]. The close association of these two common metabolic disorders has been referred to as "diabesity" [65]. Adipocytes are not merely a site for storage of energy in the form of triglycerides, but also a source of many adipokines [63] that have effects on many peripheral tissues, including skeletal muscles and liver. As body weight increases, there is expansion of the adipose tissue mass, particularly visceral intra-abdominal adipose tissue, resulting in, not only excessive free fatty acids release, but also altered release of these adipokines [66]. Increased release of various inflammatory cytokines, such as tumor necrosis factor-α (TNF-α), IL-6, MCP-1 and resistin; mainly from visceral fat and leptin; mainly from subcutaneous fat, together with decreased release of adiponectin contribute to the whole body insulin resistance [67]. Figure (3) shows how inflammation contributes to develop insulin resistance and type 2 diabetes mellitus.

The inflammation is triggered in the adipose tissue by macrophages, which form ring-like structures surrounding dead adipocytes. As adipose tissue expands during the development of obesity, certain regions become hypoperfused, leading to adipocyte microhypoxia and cell death. Adipocyte hypoxia and death trigger a series of proinflammatory program, which in turn recruit new macrophages. Another proposed mechanism is the activation of inflammatory pathway by oxidative stress. Hyperglycemia and high fat diet have been shown to increase ROS production, via multiple pathways; such as NADPH oxidase activation, which in turn activates nuclear factor-κB, triggering inflammatory response in adipose tissue [68].

TNF-α, resistin, IL-6 and other cytokines appear to participate in the induction and maintenance of the chronic low-grade inflammatory state; which is one of the hallmarks of obesity and type 2 diabetes [69]. IL-6 may interfere with insulin signaling, inhibit lipoprotein lipase activity and increase concentrations of non-esterified fatty acids (NEFA), contributing to dyslipidemia and insulin resistance [70]. In addition, IL-6 stimulates the secretion of further proinflammatory cytokines; such as IL-1 and increases the hepatic production of CRP, thus explaining its increase in the metabolic syndrome and diabetes[71].

C-reactive protein (CRP), monocyte chemoattractant protein-1 (MCP-1) and other chemokines have essential roles in the recruitment and activation of macrophages in the adipose tissue and in the initiation of inflammation [69, 72]. CRP activation of monocytes increases the expression of Ccr2, the receptor for MCP-1[72]. Overexpression of MCP-1 causes inhibition of Akt and tyrosine phosphorylation in liver and skeletal muscle, which contributes to insulin resistance [73, 74]. This demonstrates a clear association between increased levels of MCP-1 and CRP with the decreased insulin sensitivity and increased vascular inflammation [75], explaining the increased risk of atherosclerosis, cardiovascular disease and stroke in diabetic patients [76, 77].

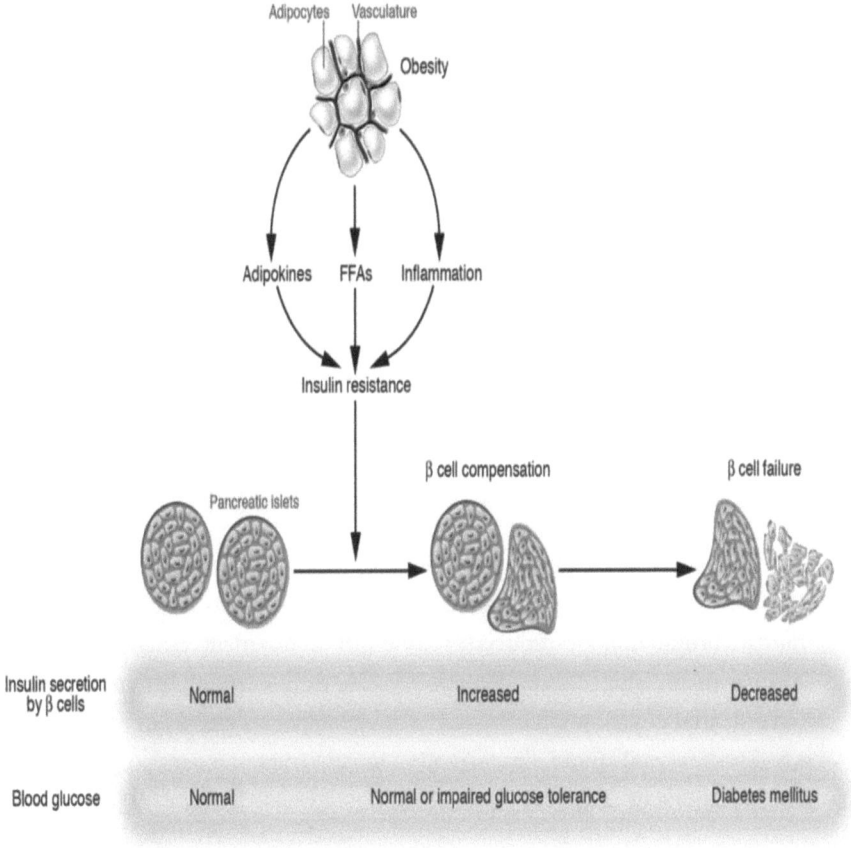

Figure (3): Development of type 2 diabetes; insulin resistance that precedes the development of hyperglycemia is associated with obesity and is induced by adipokines, FFAs, and chronic inflammation in adipose tissue. Pancreatic β-cells compensate for insulin resistance by hypersecretion of insulin. However, at some point, β-cell compensation is followed by β-cell failure and diabetes ensues [63].

This state of proatherogenesis and low-grade inflammation is known to cause induction of inducible nitric oxide synthase (iNOS), increasing nitric oxide production [78]. Nitric oxide (NO) is a free radical, known to act as a biological messenger in mammals. It has a dual role as a mediator of physiological and pathophysiological processes.

In pancreatic islets, excess NO is produced on exposure to cytokines, which mediates β-cell injury and leads to diabetes mellitus. Nitric oxide can also combine with oxygen to produce potent cellular killers, such as the highly toxic hydroxyl radical (OH·) and peroxynitrite (ONOO⁻). In diabetes mellitus, there is increased breakdown of NO by superoxide, resulting in the excessive formation of peroxynitrite, a potent oxidant that can attack many types of biological molecules. High levels of peroxynitrite cause initation of lipid peroxidation, sulfhydryl oxidation, nitration of some amino acids, direct DNA damage and oxidation of antioxidants [3].

Oxidative stress in diabetes mellitus

Oxidative stress refers to a situation of a serious imbalance between free radical-generating and radical-scavenging systems; i.e. increased free radical production or reduced activity of antioxidant defenses or both, leading to potential tissue damage [79]. There is currently great interest in the potential contribution of reactive oxygen species (ROS) in pathogenesis of diabetes and more importantly in the development of secondary complications of diabetes [80].

Free radical species include a variety of highly reactive molecules, such as ROS and reactive nitrogen species (RNS). ROS include free radicals such as superoxide ($O_2^{·-}$), hydroxyl (OH·), peroxyl ($RO_2^·$), hydroperoxyl ($HRO_2^{·-}$), as well as non-radical species such as hydrogen peroxide (H_2O_2) and hypochlorous acid (HOCl). RNS include free radicals like nitric oxide (NO·) and nitrogen dioxide ($NO_2^{·-}$), as well as non-radicals such as peroxynitrite (ONOO⁻), nitrous oxide (HNO_2) and alkyl peroxynitrates (RONOO) [81]. Production of one ROS or RNS may lead to the production of others through radical chain reactions [82]. Of these reactive molecules; $O_2^{·-}$, NO· and ONOO⁻ are the most widely studied species, as they play important roles in diabetic complications [83].

To avoid free radical overproduction, antioxidants are synthesized to neutralize free radicals. Antioxidants include a manifold of enzymes, such as superoxide dismutase (SOD), catalase, glutathione peroxidase and glutathione reductase, as well as many non-enzymatic antioxidants as vitamin A, C and E [84]. This is shown in Figure (4).

Free radicals, at physiological levels, play a key role in defense mechanisms as seen in phagocytosis and neutrophil function. They are also involved in gene transcription and, to some extent, acts as signaling molecules. However, excess generation of free radicals in oxidative stress has pathological consequences, including damage to nucleic acid, proteins and lipids, causing tissue injury and cell death [83].

Oxidative damage to DNA, lipids and proteins

1- Nucleic acid:

The hydroxyl radical is known to react with all components of the DNA molecule, damaging both the purine and pyrimidine bases and the deoxyribose backbone, causing base degeneration, single strand breakage and cross-linking to proteins. The most extensively studied DNA lesion is the formation of 8-OH-Guanine. Permanent modification of genetic material, resulting from these oxidative damage incidents, represents the first step involved in mutagenesis, carcinogenesis and ageing [85, 86].

2- Proteins:

Collectively, ROS can lead to oxidation of the side chain of amino acids residues of proteins, particularly methionine and cysteine residues, forming protein-protein cross-linkages and oxidation of the protein backbone [87], resulting in protein fragmentation, denaturation, inactivation, altered electrical charge and increased susceptibility to proteolysis [88]. The concentration of carbonyl groups is a good measure of ROS-mediated protein oxidation [89].

3- Membrane lipids:

ROS attack polyunsaturated fatty acids (PUFAs) of phospholipids in the cell membranes, which are extremely sensitive to oxidation because of double and single bonds arrangement [90]. The removal of a hydrogen atom leaves behind an unpaired electron on the carbon atom to which it was originally attached. The resulting carbon-centered lipid radical can have several fates, but the most likely one is to undergo molecular rearrangement, followed by reaction with O_2 to give a peroxyl radical, which are capable of abstracting hydrogen from adjacent fatty acid side chains and so propagating the chain reaction of lipid peroxidation. Hence, a single initiation event can result in conversion of hundreds of fatty acid side chains into lipid hydroperoxides [91]. Further decomposition of these lipid hydroperoxides produces toxic aldehydes; in particular 4-hydroxynonenal and malondialdehyde [92].

The occurrence of lipid peroxidation in biological membranes causes impairment of membrane functioning, changes in fluidity, inactivation of membrane-bound receptors and enzymes, and increased non-specific permeability to ions [93]. Thus, lipid peroxidation in-vivo has been implicated as the underlying mechanisms in numerous disorders and diseases, such as cardiovascular diseases, atherosclerosis, liver cirrhosis, cancer, neurological disorders, diabetes mellitus, rheumatoid arthritis and aging [89].

Malondialdehyde (MDA) is a major highly toxic by-product formed by PUFAs peroxidation. MDA can react both irreversibly and reversibly with proteins, DNA and phospholipids, resulting in profound mutagenic and carcinogenic effects [92, 94]. The determination of plasma, urine or other tissue MDA concentrations using thiobarbituric acid (TBA reaction) continues to be widely used as a marker of oxidative stress, as its level correlates with the extent of lipid peroxidation [95].

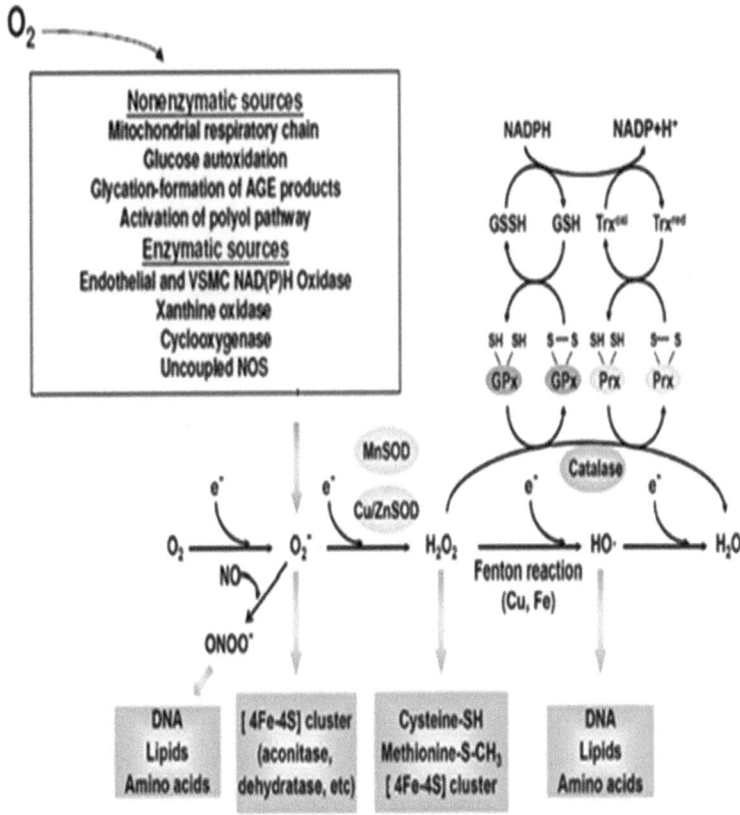

Figure (4): The cellular origins of reactive oxygen species, their targets and antioxidant systems [68, 83].

Sources of oxidative stress in diabetes

Multiple sources of oxidative stress in diabetes including enzymatic, non-enzymatic and mitochondrial pathways have been reported [81].

Enzymatic sources of augmented generation of reactive species in diabetes include NOS, NAD(P)H oxidase and xanthine oxidase. If NOS lacks its substrate L-arginine or one of its cofactors, NOS may produce $O_2^{\cdot-}$ instead of $NO^{\cdot}$ and this is referred to as the uncoupled state of NOS. NAD(P)H oxidase is a membrane associated enzyme that consists of five subunits and is a major source of $O_2^{\cdot-}$ production [81]. There is plausible evidence that protein kinase C (PKC), which is stimulated in diabetes via multiple mechanisms, activates NAD(P)H oxidase [82].

Non-enzymatic sources of oxidative stress originate from hyperglycemia, which can directly increase ROS generation. Glucose can undergo auto-oxidation and generate $OH^{\cdot}$ radicals. In addition, glucose reacts with proteins in a non-enzymatic manner, leading to the development of Amadori products followed by formation of advanced glycation endproducts (AGEs). ROS is generated at multiple steps during this process [96]. Once AGEs are formed, they bind to various receptors termed RAGE and this step is also generating ROS [97]. Moreover, cellular hyperglycemia in diabetes leads to the depletion of NADPH, through the polyol pathway, resulting in enhanced production of $O_2^{\cdot-}$ [98].

The mitochondrial respiratory chain is another source of non-enzymatic generation of reactive species. During the oxidative phosphorylation process, electrons are transferred from electron carriers NADH and $FADH_2$, through four complexes in the inner mitochondrial membrane, to oxygen, generating ATP and $O_2^{\cdot-}$, which is immediately eliminated by natural defense [83]. However, in the diabetic cells, more glucose is oxidized by Krebs cycle, which pushes more NADH and $FADH_2$ into the electron transport chain (ETC) thereby overwhelming complex III of ETC, where the transfer of electrons is blocked. Thus, the generated electrons are directly donated to molecular oxygen, one at a time, generating excessive superoxide [57]. Therefore in diabetes, electron transfer and oxidative phosphorylation are uncoupled, resulting in excessive $O_2^{\cdot-}$ formation and inefficient ATP synthesis [99].

Antioxidants

Reactive oxygen species can be eliminated by a number of antioxidant defense mechanisms, which involve both enzymatic and non-enzymatic strategies. They work in synergy with each other and against different types of free radicals [100]. Hyperglycemia not only engenders free radicals, but also impairs the endogenous antioxidant defense system and causes inflammation in many ways in diabetes mellitus [101], Figure (5). Decreases in the activities of SOD, catalase and glutathione peroxidase; decreased levels of glutathione and elevated concentrations of thiobarbituric acid reactants are consistently observed in diabetic patients and in experimentally-induced diabetes [100].

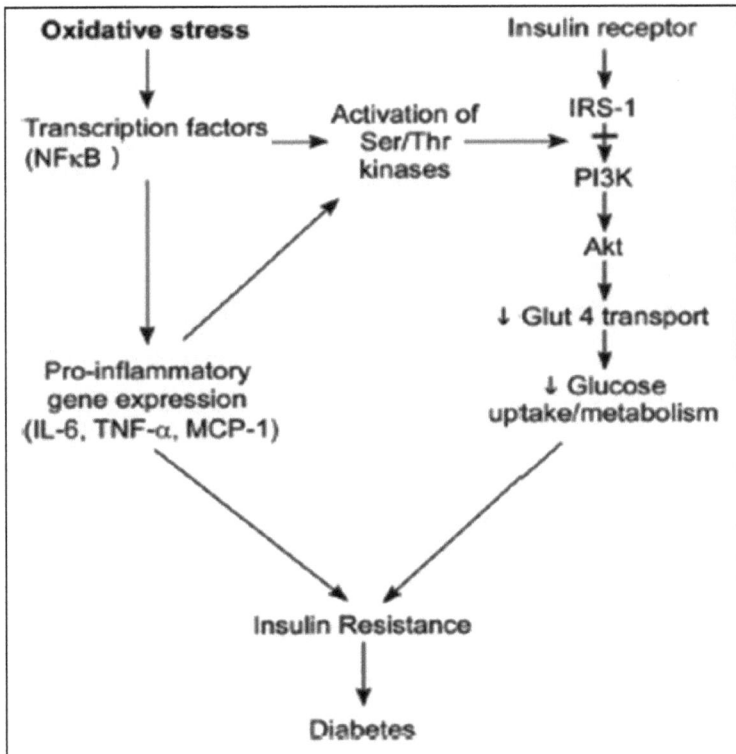

Figure (5): Schematic of the effects of chronic oxidative stress on the insulin signaling pathway [102]

I- Enzymatic antioxidants

- **Superoxide dismutase (SOD)**

Isoforms of SOD are variously located within the cell. Cu/Zn-SOD is found in both the cytoplasm and the nucleus. Mn-SOD is confined to the mitochondria, but can be released into the extracellular space [100]. SOD converts superoxide anion radicals produced in the body to hydrogen peroxide, which is then detoxified to water either by catalase or by glutathione peroxidase in the lysosomes and mitochondria, respectively[96], thereby reducing the likelihood of superoxide anion interacting with nitric oxide to form reactive peroxynitrite [100]. However, H_2O_2 can also be converted to the highly reactive $OH^.$ radical in the presence of transition elements like iron and copper [103].

II- Non-enzymatic antioxidants

1- Vitamins

Vitamins A, C and E are diet-derived and detoxify free radicals directly. They also interact in recycling processes to generate their reduced forms. α-tocopherol is reconstituted, when ascorbic acid recycles the tocopherol radical generating dihydroascorbic acid, which is recycled by glutathione [100].

Vitamin E, a fat soluble vitamin, reacts directly with peroxyl and superoxide radicals to protect membranes from lipid peroxidation [100]. It exists in eight different forms, of which α-tocopherol is the most active form in humans. Hydroxyl radical reacts with tocopherol forming a stabilized phenolic radical, which is reduced back to the phenol by ascorbate and NAD(P)H dependent reductase enzymes [96]. The deficiency of vitamin E is concurrent with increased peroxides and aldehydes in many tissues. However, there have been conflicting reports about vitamin E levels in diabetic animals and human subjects that its plasma and/or tissue levels are reported to be unaltered, increased or decreased in diabetes [100].

Vitamin C, ascorbic acid, is an important potent water soluble antioxidant vitamin in human plasma, acting as an electron donor; it is capable of scavenging oxygen-derived free radicals and sparing other endogenous antioxidants from consumption [104]. It can increase NO production in endothelial cells by stabilizing NOS cofactor tetrahydrobiopterin (BH4)[96]. Vitamin C itself is oxidized to dehydroascorbate, which is considered as a marker of oxidative stress, as in smoking and diabetes mellitus [105]. Plasma and tissue levels of vitamin C are 40–50% lower in diabetic compared with non-diabetic subjects [106].

2- Coenzyme Q_{10} (CoQ_{10})

It is an endogenously synthesized lipid soluble antioxidant that acts as an electron carrier in the complex II of the mitochondrial electron transport chain and in higher concentrations, it scavenges $O_2^{.-}$ and improves endothelial dysfunction in diabetes [83, 96].

3- α-Lipoic acid

It is an antioxidant, which can exert beneficial effects in both aqueous and lipid environments. α-lipoic acid is reduced to another active compound dihydrolipoate, which is able to regenerate other antioxidants, such as vitamin C, vitamin E and reduced glutathione through redox cycling [83, 96].

4- Trace elements

Selenium, an essential trace element, is involved in the complex defense system against oxidative stress through selenium-dependent glutathione peroxidases and other selenoproteins [107]. It has insulin-mimetic properties on glucose metabolism both in-vitro and in-vivo, by stimulating the tyrosine kinases involved in the insulin signaling cascade[108]. Within the context of diabetes mellitus, controversially data on selenium levels in biological fluids can be found. Lower, similar and even higher selenium levels were reported in diabetic patients with respect to healthy subjects [109].

Zinc, magnesium and chromium are of special interest. Severe Zn deficiency is not frequent but concerns have been raised about Zn levels in diabetic patients. Some studies have reported Zn deficiency in type 2 diabetes, others failed to find significant differences with healthy subjects [110]. Low magnesium levels have been associated with increased severity of type 2 diabetes, whereas controversy exists about the importance of hypomagnesaemia in pre-diabetic states[110]. Previous studies also reported that diabetic patients have a significantly lower plasma chromium levels with higher urinary levels than in healthy subjects. This combination of abnormalities suggests a chronic renal loss of chromium [111].

Vanadium compounds are one of the most studied substances for the long-term treatment of diabetes. Vanadium exhibits insulin-mimetic effects in-vitro and in the streptozotocin diabetic rat with some insulin-enhancing effects [112].

5- Glutathione

Glutathione (γ-glutamyl-L-cysteinylglycine, GSH), Figure (6), is a small intracellular ubiquitous tripeptide, which is a sulfhydryl (SH) antioxidant, antitoxin and enzyme cofactor [113], present in both prokaryotes and eukaryotes [114]. Being water soluble, it is found mainly in the cell cytosol and other aqueous phases of the living system [113].

Glutathione antioxidant system predominates among other antioxidants systems due to its very high reduction potential and high intracellular concentrations compared to other antioxidants in tissues. Glutathione is found almost exclusively in its thiol-reduced active form (GSH), comprises 90% of the total low molecular weight thiol in the body [115]. GSH often attains millimolar levels inside cells, especially highly concentrated in the liver and in lens, spleen, kidney, erythrocytes and leukocytes, however its plasma concentration is in micromolar range [116].

Glutathione is an essential cofactor for antioxidant enzymes, namely the GSH peroxidases, which serve to detoxify hydrogen peroxide and other peroxides generated in water phase as well as the cell membranes and other lipophilic cell phases by reacting them with GSH, which then becomes in the oxidized form (GSSG). The recycling of GSSG to GSH is accomplished mainly by the enzyme glutathione reductase using the coenzyme NADPH as its source of electrons. Therefore NADPH, coming mainly from the pentose phosphate shunt, is the predominant source of GSH reducing power [117]. Moreover, GSH is an essential component of the glyoxalase enzyme system, which is responsible for catabolism of the highly reactive aldehydes; methylglyoxal and glyoxal. It can also bind to these aldehydes, causing them to be excreted in bile and urine [115]. These effects have particular implications for preventive health, as lipid peroxidation has been found to contribute to the development of many chronic diseases in humans.

The ratio of reduced to oxidized glutathione (GSH/GSSG) within cells is often used as a measure of cellular toxicity or vice versa as a predictor of the antioxidative capacity and redox state of the cells [114]. GSH in the body is synthesized mostly de-novo, with cysteine being the limiting amino acid, so increasing cysteine supply is necessary to raise GSH synthesis and concentration. GSH may be a good reservoir for cysteine, as its concentration in tissues is 5-7 times higher than free cysteine [118].

$$\underset{HO}{\overset{O}{\underset{\|}{C}}}-CH-CH_2-CH_2-\underset{\overset{\|}{O}}{C}-NH-\underset{\overset{|}{CH_2}}{\overset{|}{CH}}-\underset{\overset{\|}{O}}{C}-NH-CH_2-\underset{OH}{\overset{O}{\underset{\|}{C}}}$$

γ-carboxyl linkage

γ-glutamyl   cysteinyl   glycine

Figure (6): Structure of GSH (γ-glutamylcysteinyl glycine), where the N-terminal glutamate and cysteine are linked by the γ-carboxyl group of glutamate [119].

GSH makes major contributions to the recycling of other antioxidants that have become oxidized such as α-tocopherol, vitamin C and perhaps also the carotenoids [117]. Moreover, GSH is important in the synthesis and repair of DNA, as it is required in the conversion of ribonucleotides to deoxyribonucleotides [120].

A major function of GSH is the detoxification of xenobiotics and/or their metabolites. It is also involved in maintaining the essential thiol status of many important enzymes and proteins [117]. It participates in some cellular functions as amino acid translocation across the cell membrane [121] and folding of newly synthesized proteins [122]. In addition, GSH is essential for the proliferation, growth, differentiation and activation of immune cells[117] and is implicated in the modulation of cell death (cellular apoptosis and necrosis) [123].

Some oxidative stressors are known for their ability to deplete GSH. These include smoking, alcohol intake, some over the counter drugs (as acetaminophen), household chemicals, strenuous aerobic exercise, dietary deficiency of methionine (an essential amino acid and GSH precursor), ionizing radiation, tissue injury, surgery, trauma, bacterial or viral infections (as HIV-1) and environmental toxins [117].

GSH reduction has been associated with the pathogenesis of a variety of diseases; therefore, systemic GSH status could serve as an index of general health.

Glutathione in liver diseases

GSH depletion is involved in liver injury and enhanced morbidity related to liver hypofunction. Studies had been demonstrated a decrease in plasma and liver GSH, increase in GSSG and a significant decrease in cysteine present in cirrhotic patients, chronic alcoholic and non-alcoholic liver disease (fatty liver, acute and chronic hepatitis); as compared with the healthy subjects [117].

Glutathione in immunity and HIV disease

Adequate GSH is essential for mounting successful immune responses when the host is immunologically challenged. Healthy humans with relatively low lymphocyte GSH were found to have significantly lower CD4 counts [117]. It was postulated that GSH deficiency could lead to the progression of immune dysfunction, weight loss, cachexia and wasting syndrome, which are known AIDS stigmas. GSH depletion is also seen in many autoimmune diseases as Crohn's disease, an inflammatory immunomediated disorder, in which low GSH, elevated GSSG levels and altered GSH enzymes were found in the affected ileal zones [114].

Glutathione in diabetes mellitus

Low blood thiol status and reduced systemic GSH content were reported in diabetic and glucose intolerant patients as a result of insulin deficiency. It was reported that chronic hyperglycemia resulted in enhanced apoptosis in human endothelial cells, which was attenuated by insulin due to its ability to induce glutamate cysteine ligase expression [119]. Platelets from diabetics have lower GSH levels and make excess thromboxane (TxA2), thus having a lowered threshold for aggregation. This may contribute to the increased atherosclerosis seen in the diabetic population[117].

Furthermore, glutathione deficiency is associated with aging and many other diseases as neurodegenerative diseases, including Parkinson's disease, schizophrenia and Alzheimer's disease; atherosclerosis and cardiovascular diseases; human pancreatic inflammatory diseases and metal storage diseases as Wilson's disease [117, 124].

Strategies for repleting cellular glutathione

In light of the copious evidence supporting the importance of GSH for homeostasis, and for resistance to toxic attack, as well as the contribution of its deficiency in many diseases, a number of researchers had been stimulated to find new potential approaches and methods for maintaining or restoring GSH levels [125]. Optimizing GSH would likely augment antioxidant defenses and stabilize or raise the cell's threshold for susceptibility to toxic attack [117].

- **Oral glutathione**

Oral GSH was reported to replete GSH in subjects with depleted GSH but not healthy ones. Intact GSH can be absorbed slowly by intestinal lumen enterocytes and epithelial cells, such as lung alveolar cells; thus intact GSH can be also delivered directly into the lungs as an aerosol [117]. Circulating GSH is safe and soluble in plasma. It reacts only slowly with oxygen and is less susceptible to auto-oxidative degradation. However, currently, the use of GSH as a therapeutic agent is limited by its unfavorable pharmacokinetic properties. GSH has a short half-life in human plasma and difficulty in crossing cell membranes, so administration of high doses is necessary to reach a therapeutic value [125], which will not be a particularly cost-effective way to accomplish GSH repletion.

- **L-cysteine**

It is a sulfur containing semi-essential amino acid, as humans can synthesize it from the essential amino acid methionine only to a limited and generally not sufficient extent [126]. Its chemical structure is illustrated in Figure (7). One important function of L-cysteine is being a precursor that limits the synthesis of glutathione. It also serves as a very important precursor for synthesis of proteins, coenzyme A and inorganic sulphate [127].

Cysteine is catabolized in the gastrointestinal tract and plasma [128], so it is relatively unstable in the blood. When substituted into the diet in place of the total protein allowance, it can replete GSH [117].

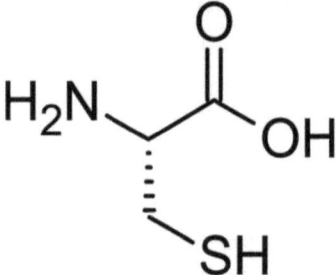

Figure (7): Chemical structure of L-cysteine [115]

Biosynthesis

In animals, L-cysteine is synthesized from L-methionine and L-serine via trans-sulfurtion reaction [127]. The sulfur is derived from methionine, which is converted to homocysteine through the intermediate S-adenosylmethionine. Cystathionine β-synthase then combines homocysteine and serine to form the asymmetrical thioether, cystathionine. The enzyme cystathionine γ-lyase converts the cystathionine into cysteine and α-ketobutyrate [129]. This is shown in Figure (8).

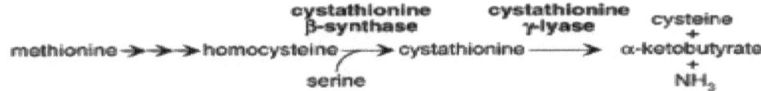

Figure (8): The transsulfuration pathway in animals. The first three reactions involve methyl group transfer via S-adenosylmethionine [129].

Biological functions of L-cysteine

The chemical structure of cysteine contains a free sulfhydryl group, which is the reactive entity that contributes to many of cysteine's biological activity; serving as a nucleophile with susceptibility to be oxidized to the disulfide derivative cystine [130].

As a moderately powerful redox pair, cysteine and its disulfide partner cystine have an important physiological function as antioxidants. Cysteine's antioxidant properties are typically expressed in the glutathione, where the free SH group of cysteine within glutathione confers its functional properties. Cysteine and glutathione form a major part of the endogenous thiol pool that reacts with the vasoregulatory molecule NO to form nitrosothiol, which acts as NO-carrier molecules, stabilizing this normally volatile molecule. S-nitrosothiols have potent relaxant activity, antiaggregatory and anti-inflammatory functions. They have greater half-lives than free NO and are more resistant than free NO to degradation by superoxide. In this way, nitrosothiol increases the bioavailability of NO and potentiates its effects [115]. All actions of cysteine and GSH are shown in Figure (9).

Cysteine is a component of many structural and functional proteins. It is able to stabilize protein structures by forming disulfide covalent cross-links, which add stability to the three-dimensional structures of protein, increase the rigidity of proteins, affect their susceptibility to denaturation and provide proteolytic resistance [115, 131]. The precise location of cysteine within a protein also plays a direct role in the protein's function. For

33

example, cysteine is found at the active site of several enzymes, including eNOS; regulating its catalytic activity [115].

Proteins containing cysteine, such as metallothionein, can bind to heavy metals tightly because of the high affinity of thiol group to these metals; thus cobalt, cupper, inorganic arsenic and selenium toxicities can be ameliorated by oral cysteine ingestion[132]. L-cysteine has been proposed as a preventative or antidote for some of the negative effects of alcohol, including liver damage and hangover. It counteracts the poisonous effects of acetaldehyde; the major by-product of alcohol metabolism, by supporting its conversion into the relatively harmless acetic acid [133]. Aside from its oxidation to cystine, cysteine participates in numerous post-translational modifications[134].

Cysteine and insulin resistance

An early study demonstrated that cysteine has an insulin-like action, promoting the entry of glucose into adipose cells, mediated by its free SH group. Cysteine has been subsequently shown to increase the levels of GLUT3 and GLUT4, with a marked enhancement of glucose uptake, in mouse muscle and human neuroblastoma cells [135]. Moreover, Cysteine may improve glucose metabolism by preventing oxidative or nitrosative inhibition of the glycolytic enzymes glyceraldehyde-3-phosphate dehydrogenase and glucose-6- phosphate dehydrogenase [115].

In cultured adipocytes, it was demonstrated that cysteine supplementation reverses the increased intracellular oxidative stress, after AGE-RAGE interaction, which causes a decrease in glucose uptake [136] and also prevents the methylglyoxal induced decrease in IRS-1 tyrosine phosphorylation and PI3K activity that impair insulin signaling [137]. This is illustrated in Figure (10).

It was also reported that cysteine analogues potentiate the glucose-induced insulin release in pancreatic islets isolated from female Wistar rats[138]. Dietary intake of whey protein and α-lactoalbumin (cysteine-rich proteins) lowers the oxidative stress and insulin resistance induced by sucrose in rats [139]. Other studies have reported that N-acetylcysteine supplementation reduces fructose-induced insulin resistance in rats [140] and also improves insulin sensitivity in women with polycystic ovaries [141].

Other effects of L-cysteine

1- L-cysteine administration prevents liver fibrosis by direct inhibition of activated hepatic stellate cells proliferation and transformation [142]. It also shows a cytoprotective effect against carbon tetrachloride (CCl_4)-induced hepatotoxicity by reversal of CCl_4 induced lactate dehydrogenase release and decreased cellular thiols, mainly glutathione [143].

2- Previous clinical studies suggest that the acquired immunodeficiency syndrome (AIDS) may be the consequence of a virus-induced cysteine deficiency. HIV-infected persons were found to have abnormally high TNF-α and IL-2 receptor alpha-chain. All the corresponding genes are associated with NF-κB, whose transcription is negatively regulated by cysteine or cysteine derivatives, thus they may be considered as adjuvant therapy for the treatment of patients with HIV-1 infection [144, 145].

Side effects of L-cysteine

Gastrointestinal problems as indigestion, flatulence, diarrhea, nausea and vomiting are the main side effects of L-cysteine. Allergic reactions, include itching and facial swelling, are another possible side effects. Copious amount of water should be taken with cysteine to prevent cystine renal stones formation. It was showed by in-vitro studies that cysteine mimics many of the chemical properties of homocysteine, which is known to increase the risk of the cardiovascular diseases [146].

N-acetylcysteine (NAC)

N-acetyl-L-cysteine is a cysteine precursor that is rapidly absorbed and converted to circulating cysteine by deacetylation. It is used as an antioxidant and as a mucolytic due to its ability to break disulphide bonds in the mucous. It has liver protecting effects, so it is a well-established antidote for acetaminophen overdose [147]. It also has antimutagenic and anticarcinogenic properties. In addition, NAC can prevent apoptosis and promote cell survival, a concept useful for treating certain degenerative diseases [148].

NAC can scavenge ROS and increase depleted glutathione levels. Activation of redox-sensitive NF-κB in response to a variety of signals (IL-1, TNF-α and ROS) can be also inhibited by NAC. NAC can interfere with cell adhesion, smooth muscle cell proliferation, stability of rupture-prone atherosclerotic plaques in the cardiovascular system, reduce lung inflammation and prolong survival of transplants [148].

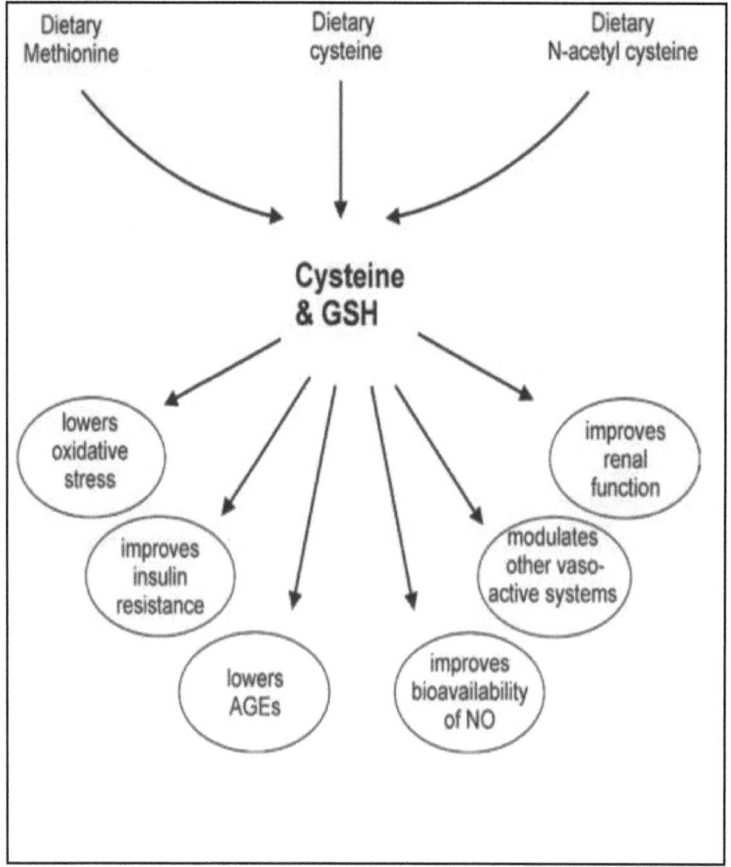

Figure (9): Sources and actions of cysteine and glutathione (GSH) [115].

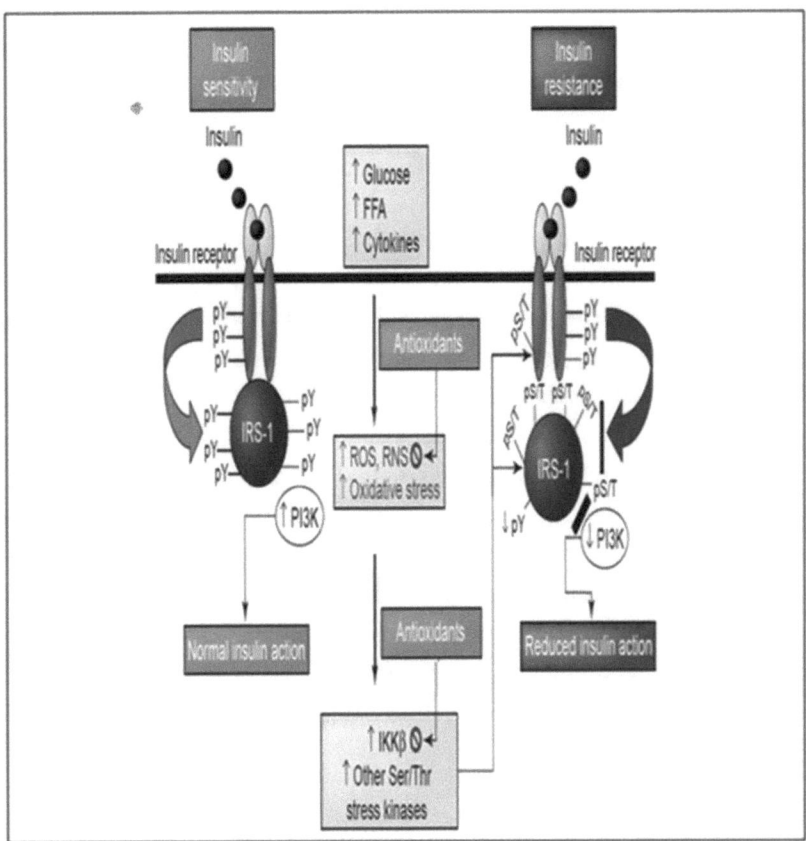

Figure (10): The role of serine kinase activation in oxidative stress-induced insulin resistance and the protective effect of some antioxidants by preserving the intracellular redox balance[149].

Management of diabetes mellitus

I- Non-pharmacological management of diabetes

Lifestyle modifications are the cornerstone of management of diabetes mellitus and include the prescription of a healthy diet, regular exercise, management of stress and avoidance of tobacco [150].

1-Diet

The aims of dietary management are to achieve and maintain ideal body weight, euglycemia and desirable lipid profile, prevent and postpone complications related to diabetes and provide optimal nutrition during pregnancy, lactation, growth, old age and associated conditions, such as hypertension and catabolic illnesses [151]. However, there is no single description for diet composition that can achieve these goals in all patients. Thus, the dietary recommendations should be individualized according to the person's ethnicity, cultural and family background, personal preferences and associated co-morbid conditions [150]. Diet, that contains 60% carbohydrates, high dietary fiber, low to moderate dietary fat and moderate high biological value proteins as well as vitamins and minerals; especially chromium, vitamin E and C, is considered proper for management of diabetic patients [152].

2- Physical activity

Exercise program should be individualized according to patient's capacity and disabilities. Diabetic patient must wear appropriate footwear. It should also be noted that poorly controlled patients may develop hyperglycemia during exercise, whereas patients treated with insulin and insulin secretagogues could develop hypoglycemia [153].

The best form of exercise recommended to diabetic is a stepwise increase of aerobic exercises. There are several benefits from a regular exercise schedule. These include reduction of hypertension and weight, increase in bone density, improvement in insulin sensitivity, cardiovascular function and lipid profile (reduces serum triglycerides and increases HDL-C), as well as improvement in the sense of physical and mental well-being and the overall quality of life [152].

3- Stress management

Diagnosis of diabetes mellitus is a stressful situation in life of an individual and appropriate management; requires an approach that includes behavioural modification to develop positive attitude and healthy life style. A satisfactory treatment plan should include special attention to person with diabetes, quality of life, coping skills, optimal family support and a healthy workplace environment. Appropriate support and counseling is an essential component of the management at the time of diagnosis and throughout life[150].

II- Pharmacological management of type 2 diabetes mellitus

A- Antidiabetic agents

Even when non-pharmacological measures are successfully implemented, the progressive natural history of the disease dictates that the majority of patients will later require pharmacologic therapy, and this should be introduced promptly if the glycemic target is not met or not maintained. Preserving β-cell function and mass are important considerations in maintaining long-term glycemic control. If β-cell function deteriorates beyond the capacity of oral agents to provide adequate glycemic control, then the introduction of insulin should not be delayed[154].

Terminology within the field of antidiabetic agents may simplify the usage of the different agents. Hypoglycemic agents have the capacity to lower blood glucose below normal level to the extent of frank hypoglycemia (e.g. sulfonylureas). Antihyperglycemic agents (euglycemic agents) can reduce hyperglycemia, but when acting alone they do not have the capability to lower blood glucose below normoglycemia to the extent of frank hypoglycemia (e.g. metformin, thiazolidinediones, gliptins, α-glucosidase inhibitors) [154].

They are classified into:

- **Oral antidiabetic agents:**
  - Insulin sensitizers:
    - Biguanides, including metformin
    - Thiazolidinediones or glitazones, including rosiglitazone and pioglitazone
  - Insulin secretagogues:
    - Sulfonylureas, including gliclazide, glipizide, glimepiride and glibenclamide
    - Meglitinides (non-sulfonylurea secretagogues) including nateglinide and repaglinide
  - Alpha-glucosidase inhibitors including acarbose, miglitol and voglibose

- **Novel treatments:** (oral and non-insulin parenteral agents)
    - Gliptins, including sitagliptin and vildagliptin
    - Glucagon-like peptide-1 receptor agonist, including exenatide and liraglutide
    - Amylin and amylin analogs, including pramlintide
    - Rimonabant

- **New experimental agents**

1. Insulin sensitizers

1.1. Biguanides

The history of biguanides stems from a guanidine-rich herb Galega officinalis (goat's rue or French lilac) that was used as a traditional treatment for diabetes in Europe because of its glucose lowering effect [154, 155]. Its structural formula is illustrated in Figure (11).

Several guanidine derivatives were adopted for the treatment of diabetes in the 1920s. These agents all disappeared as insulin became available, but three biguanides – metformin, phenformin and buformin – were introduced in the late 1950s [155]. However, phenformin and buformin were withdrawn in many countries in the late 1970s because of a high incidence of lactic acidosis [156]. Metformin remained and was introduced into the USA in 1995 and since then it became most widely prescribed first line antidiabetic agent worldwide [157].

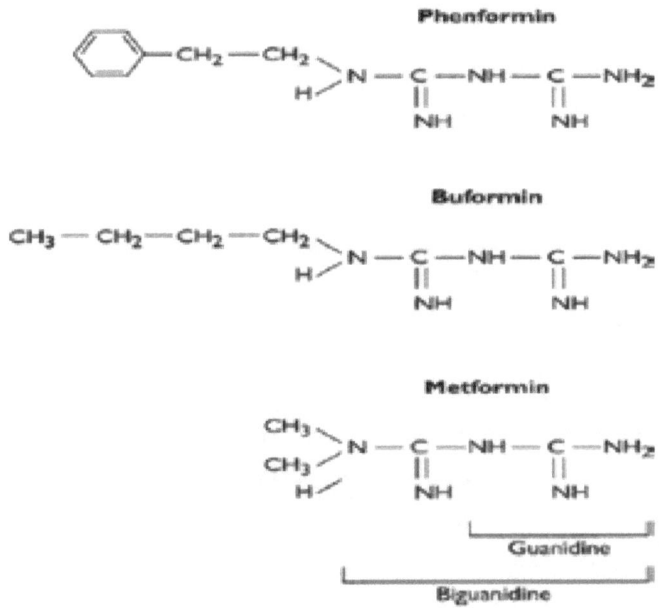

Figure (11): Chemical structure of biguanides [158].

Pharmacological effects of metformin

1- Antihyperglycemic effect

Metformin exerts a range of actions that counter insulin resistance and decrease hyperglycemia by reducing fasting and postprandial blood glucose[159]. The glucose-lowering efficacy of metformin requires a presence of at least some insulin because metformin does not mimic or activate the genomic effects of insulin. The precise mechanisms through which metformin exerts its glucose lowering effects are not entirely understood. However, its primary mode of action appears to be increasing hepatic insulin sensitivity, resulting in decreased hepatic glucose output through suppression of gluconeogenesis and glycogenolysis. Metformin may also modestly augment glucose uptake in peripheral tissues, increase fatty acid oxidation and increase glucose metabolism in the splanchnic bed. Metformin's molecular effects appear to be at least in part mediated by adenosine monophosphate-activated protein kinase (AMPK), but it is unclear if this pathway represents the drug's specific or unique target [160]. AMPK activation determines a wide variety of physiological effects, including increased fatty acid oxidation and enhanced glucose uptake by skeletal muscle by increasing translocation of GLUT1 and insulin-sensitive glucose transporters, GLUT4, into the cell membrane [161]. Administration of metformin to obese subjects was also found to increase levels of active GLP-1 after a glucose load, this phenomenon appears to occur through mechanisms other than DPP-4 inhibition; and may instead be due to direct stimulation of GLP-1 secretion or a reduction in DPP-4 secretion [160]. Interestingly, these incretin-sensitizing effects of metformin appear to be mediated by PPAR-α dependent pathway as opposed to the more commonly described AMPK activation pathway [162]. Importantly, the likelihood of hypoglycemia induced by metformin monotherapy is quite low, as the drug does not exert its effects through an increase in insulin secretion [160].

A new insight on the mechanism of action of metformin is its ability to decrease plasma glucose through the release of β-endorphin from adrenal gland, which activates peripheral opoid μ_1 receptors. β-endorphin acts as a positive regulator in glucose utilization and a negative modulator in hepatic gluconeogenesis in the insulin-deficient state. These actions are mediated by the amelioration of GLUT4 gene expression and the attenuation of raised hepatic phosphenolpyruvate carboxykinase (PEPCK) gene expression, a rate-controlling enzyme of gluconeogenesis [163].

Metformin also has cardioprotective benefits and offers some protection against vascular complications; independently of its antihyperglycemic effect [164]. It was reported that metformin is associated with a decrease in myocardial infarction due to its effect on various atherothrombotic risk markers and factors, including reduced carotid intima-media thickness, increased fibrinolysis and reduced concentrations of the anti-thrombolytic factor; plasminogen activator inhibitor-1 (PAI-1) (154).

2-Anti-inflammatory effect

Metformin also offers some protection against vascular inflammation and complications; independently of its antihyperglycemic effect (165). This may be mediated through the reduction of thrombotic factor and inflammatory markers (166).

3-Antioxidative effect

Metformin may also exert antioxidative effects, as it prevents hyperglycemia-induced PKC activation and protects against high glucose-induced oxidative stress through a mitochondrial permeability transition dependent pathway that is involved in cell death(167). This may be in relation to metformin's ability to inhibit non-toxically complex I in the mitochondrial respiratory chain (165).

Metformin is also able to react in-vitro with OH˙ radical. However, it is not a very good scavenger of ROS at molecular level. Thus, it seems that metformin exerts its in-vivo antioxidant activity by different pathways other than the simple free radical scavenging action. These pathways include increasing the antioxidant enzyme activities, decreasing the markers of lipid peroxidation (168) and inhibiting the formation of advanced glycation end products by its ability to react directly with, and neutralize, highly reactive α-dicarbonyl intermediates involved in AGEs formation, such as methylglyoxal (164). Metformin can also increase the activity of glyoxalase, an enzyme which deactivates methylglyoxal to D-lactate (164).

Pharmacokinetics of metformin

Metformin is an orally administered medication, which is 50%–60% bioavailable. Administration with food may decrease its absorption, the clinical significance of which is unknown. The drug is minimally protein-bound, and has few known drug interactions other than that known to occur with cimetidine, which increases metformin levels in plasma by up to 40%. Metformin is not metabolized prior to its complete excretion in the urine via glomerular filtration and tubular secretion. The drug has an elimination half-life of approximately 6 hours. Decreases in renal function will decrease clearance of the medication. It is generally dosed 2–3 times daily, but is available in an extended release preparation, which may be administered once a day. 85% of the maximal glucose-lowering effect is seen at a daily dose of 500 mg 3 times daily, while the most effective glucose lowering occurs with a total daily dose of 2000 mg [160].

Indications

Because metformin does not cause weight gain, it is often preferred for overweight and obese people with T2DM. It can be introduced in insulin-resistant states before the development of hyperglycemia [163]. Metformin can resume ovulation in women with anovulatory polycystic ovarian syndrome (PCOS), which is an unlicensed application of the drug in the absence of diabetes [154].

Adverse effects and contraindications

The main tolerability issue with metformin is abdominal discomfort and other gastrointestinal adverse effects, including diarrhea, nausea, vomiting, flatulence, stomach upset and metallic taste in approximately 30% of patients [169]. Anorexia and stomach fullness are likely part of the reason for weight loss, noted with metformin. These effects are often transient and can be ameliorated by taking the drug with meals and using a small initial dose, which is then gradually titrated slowly until target level of blood glucose control is attained or using extended-release preparations of metformin[170]; however, around 5% of patients cannot tolerate the drug at any dose [171]. It can reduce gastrointestinal absorption of vitamin B_{12}, which rarely causes frank anemia [172].

The most serious adverse event associated with metformin is lactic acidosis that is typically characterized by a raised blood lactate concentration, decreased arterial pH and/or bicarbonate concentration with an increased anion gap. It is rare, but about half of cases are fatal [154]. The true likelihood of lactic acidosis, occurring as a result of metformin accumulation, is unclear. However, given these concerns, the drug is contraindicated in the setting of renal dysfunction or in those at risk for lactic acidosis, such as individuals with kidney hypoperfusion due to hypotension or septicemia, congestive heart failure, chronic cardiopulmonary dysfunction, significant hepatic dysfunction or alcohol abuse. Renal function must be assessed prior to and periodically during metformin therapy, particularly in the elderly [160].

Presenting symptoms of lactic acidosis are generally non-specific (flu-like symptoms), but often include hyperventilation, malaise and abdominal discomfort. Treatment should be commenced promptly; bicarbonate remains the usual therapy. Hemodialysis to remove excess metformin can be helpful, and may assist restoration of fluid and electrolyte imbalance occurred during treatment with high dose intravenous bicarbonate [154].

Metformin also should be temporarily stopped when using intravenous radiographic contrast media or during surgery with general anaesthesia [154].

1.2. Thiazolidinediones (TZDs)

TZDs are pharmacological ligands for the nuclear receptor peroxisome proliferator- activated receptor- γ (PPAR-γ), which is highly expressed in adipose tissue and to a lesser extent in muscle, pancreatic β-cells, vascular endothelium and macrophages [173]. Therefore, thiazolidinediones can affect responsive genes at these locations, giving rise to "pleiotropic effects" [174]. Many of these genes participate in lipid and carbohydrate metabolism.

Troglitazone was the first thiazolidinedione to enter routine clinical use; however, it was associated with fatal cases of idiosyncratic hepatotoxicity and was withdrawn in 2000[175]. Two other thiazolidinediones; rosiglitazone and pioglitazone were then introduced, which did not show hepatotoxicity, indicating that troglitazone's hepatotoxicity has presumably a compound specific phenomenon [176]. However, rosiglitazone was withdrawn in 2010 from market, as the clinical investigations revealed its implication in cardiovascular side effects [177].

Mode of action

TZDs stimulate PPAR-γ, promoting differentiation of pre-adipocytes into mature adipocytes [178]; these new small adipocytes are particularly sensitive to insulin and show increased uptake of fatty acids with increased lipogenesis [179]. This, in turn, reduces circulating free fatty acids, facilitating glucose utilization and restricting fatty acid availability as a source for hepatic gluconeogenesis. By reducing circulating fatty acids, ectopic lipid deposition in muscle and liver is reduced, which further contributes to improvements of glucose metabolism. TZDs also increase glucose uptake into adipose tissue and skeletal muscle via increased availability of GLUT4 glucose transporters [154].

Pharmacokinetics

Absorption of rosiglitazone and pioglitazone is rapid and almost complete, with peak concentrations at 1-2 hours, but slightly delayed when taken with food. Both drugs are metabolized extensively by the liver and are almost completely bound to plasma proteins; but their concentrations are not sufficient to interfere with other protein-bound drugs [154].

Indications

TZDs are indicated as monotherapy in T2DM, associated with no risk for hypoglycemia development. They are often used to gain additive efficacy in combination with other antidiabetic drugs, particularly metformin in overweight patients[180]. Interestingly, because of the effects of thiazolidinediones on hepatic fat metabolism, these drugs might even be useful for the treatment of non-alcoholic steatohepatitis [181].

Adverse effects and contraindications

Fluid retention, leading to weight gain, anemia and development of heart failure as well as increased incidence of bone fractures are the major adverse effects of TZDs[153, 182].

Their use is contraindicated in patients with evidence of heart failure or pre-existing liver disease [183] and they should be used with caution in patients with osteoporosis and pre-existing macular edema [184]. A debate on the risk of tumor development upon stimulation of PPAR-γ in colonic cells has been reported; thus, familial polyposis coli is a contraindication to TZDs on the theoretical grounds [183].

2. Insulin secretagogues

2.1. Sulfonylureas

Since their introduction in the 1950s, sulfonylureas (SUs) have been used extensively as insulin secretagogues for the treatment of T2DM. Sulfonylureas were developed as structural variants of sulfonamides, after the latter were reported to cause hypoglycemia. Early sulfonylureas such as carbutamide, tolbutamide and chlorpropamide are often referred to as "first generation". These have been largely superceded by the more potent, probably safer "second generation" sulfonylureas, notably glibenclamide (glyburide), gliclazide, glipizide; and then followed by glimepiride, which is considered "third generation" of SUs [183].

Mode of action

Sulfonylureas act directly on the β-cells of the islets of Langerhans to stimulate insulin secretion. They enter β-cell and bind to the cytosolic surface of the sulfonylurea receptor 1 (SUR1), which forms part of voltage dependent K^+ ATP channels, leading to its closure and reducing the efflux of potassium, enabling membrane depolarization, which in turn opens adjacent voltage-dependent L-type calcium channels, increasing calcium influx and causing release of insulin [185]. They are ineffective in totally insulin-deficient patients, requiring about 30% of normal β-cells function for successful therapy [186]. SUs don't increase insulin formation but stimulate the release of stored insulin in response to glucose concentrations, which are below the normal threshold for glucose-stimulated insulin release (approximately 5 mmol/L), thus they are capable of causing hypoglycemia in normal and diabetic subjects [183].

Sulfonylureas appear to enhance insulin-stimulated glucose utilization in liver, muscle and adipose tissue through increasing insulin receptor number and enhancing the post-receptor complex enzyme reactions mediated by insulin [187]. They are capable of suppressing hepatic glucose production and potentiating adipose tissue glucose transport and lipogenesis, as well as skeletal muscle glucose uptake and glycogen synthesis [154]. It has been advocated that sulfonylurea drugs have extrapancreatic effects, in addition to their insulin secretory effect on pancreatic β-cells, as they effectively improve peripheral insulin resistance through activation of peroxisome proliferator-activated receptor-γ (PPAR-γ like activity) [188].

Pharmacokinetics

Sulfonylureas vary considerably in their pharmacokinetic properties, which in turn affects their clinical suitability for different patients. Longer acting sulfonylureas can be given once daily, but carry greater risk of hypoglycemia, especially those with active metabolites. Sulfonylureas are highly bound to plasma proteins, which can lead to interactions with other protein-bound drugs, such as salicylates, NSAIDs, sulfonamides and warfarin, increasing the risk of hypoglycemia [154].

Other drug interactions include:

- Interactions that increase glucose lowering effect of SUs; as with some antifungals and MAOIs by reducing hepatic metabolism and with probencid by decreasing excretion.
- Interactions that decrease glucose lowering effect of SUs; as with rifampicin and other microsomal enzyme inducers.

Indications

Sulfonylureas are widely used as monotherapy and in combination with metformin, a thiazolidinedione or an α-glucosidase inhibitor [189]. These combinations afford an additive glucose-lowering efficacy, at least initially, but increase the risk of hypoglycemia.

Adverse effects and contraindications

Weight gain, reflects the anabolic effects of increased plasma insulin concentrations. Hypoglycemia is the most common and potentially most serious adverse effect of sulfonylurea therapy. Very occasionally, sulfonylureas produce sensitivity reactions [183].

2.2. Meglitinides (short-acting prandial insulin releasers)

Nowadays, postprandial hyperglycemia is widely recognized as a central feature of early diabetes and impaired glucose tolerance (IGT). It is caused primarily by the impairment of first phase insulin secretion and its correction is important for long-term glycemic control [190]. Meglitinide analogs, known as non-sulfonylurea secretagogues, were evaluated as potential antidiabetic agents after an observation in the 1980s that meglitinide, the non-sulfonylurea moiety of glibenclamide, could stimulate insulin secretion similar to sulfonylureas. Repaglinide, which was the first approved member of this group, and nateglinide, were introduced as "prandial insulin releasers" [191].

Mode of action

Prandial insulin releasers act similar to SUs. However, they activate a different potassium channel in the pancreatic β-cell, leading to membrane depolarization and insulin release [192]. By generating a prompt increase of insulin to coincide with meal digestion; these agents help to restore partially the first phase glucose-induced insulin response that is lost in T2DM. Specifically targeting postprandial hyperglycemia might also address the vascular risk attributed to prandial glucose excursions and reduce the risk of interprandial hypoglycemia as less insulin is secreted several hours after meal [154].

Pharmacokinetics

The pharmacokinetic properties of these compounds favored a rapid but short-lived insulin secretory effect that suited administration with meals to promote prandial insulin release. Repaglinide is almost completely and rapidly absorbed with peak plasma concentrations after about 1 hour. It is quickly metabolized in the liver to inactive metabolites and rapidly eliminated in the bile with a terminal elimination half-life of 1 to 1.7 hours [193]. Taken about 15 minutes before a meal; repaglinide produces a prompt insulin response, which lasts about 3 hours, coinciding with the duration of meal digestion[183]. Repaglinide may be more suitable than nateglinide in patients with moderate renal insufficiency, where metformin and some SUs are contraindicated [183, 192].

Indications

They are theoretically safer in older adults; particularly if other agents are contraindicated because of their short half-life and lower risk of hypoglycemia; however, the need for multiple daily dosages may be a disincentive. They can be used in patients who have an allergy to SUs medication [192]. Prandial insulin releasers can be used as monotherapy in patients inadequately controlled by non-pharmacological measures or as add-ons to metformin or TZDs to produce a synergistic effect [154].

Adverse effects

Fewer and less severe hypoglycemic episodes occur with meglitinides than with sulfonylureas. They have a similar risk for weight gain as SUs [192]. Sensitivity reactions are uncommon [183].

3. α-Glucosidase inhibitors

Acarbose, the first α-glucosidase inhibitor, was introduced in the early 1990s, followed by two further agents, miglitol and voglibose [194].

Mode of action

Their mechanism of action is unique. This is the sole dug class not targeted at a specific pathophysiological defect of type 2 DM. They competitively inhibit the activity of α-glucosidase enzymes in the brush border of enterocytes lining the intestinal villi, preventing the enzymes from cleaving disaccharides and oligosaccharides into monosaccharides, the final steps of carbohydrate digestion, delaying glucose absorption. By moving glucose absorption more distally along the intestinal tract, α-glucosidase inhibitors may alter the release of glucose-dependent intestinal hormones, GIP and GLP-1, which probably reduce postprandial insulin concentrations concurrently with the attenuated rise in postprandial glucose levels [183]. Thus, α-glucosidase inhibitors can effectively reduce postprandial glucose excursions and improves glycemic control [195].

Pharmacokinetics

Acarbose is degraded by amylases in the small intestine and by intestinal bacteria; less than 2% of the unchanged drug is absorbed along with some of the intestinal degradation products. Absorbed material is mostly eliminated in the urine within 24 hours[183, 194]. Miglitol is almost completely absorbed and eliminated unchanged in the urine and faeces [194].

Indications and contraindications

α-Glucosidase inhibitors can be used rarely as monotherapy, due to comparatively mild efficacy [189], for type 2 diabetic patients with postprandial hyperglycemia but only slightly raised fasting glycemia; however, they are more commonly used as add-on to other therapies, again to target postprandial hyperglycemia [196]. They should be taken with meals; they are most effective when given with a starchy, complex digestible carbohydrate, high-fiber diet with restricted amounts of glucose and sucrose [154].

α-Glucosidase inhibitors are contraindicated for patients with a history of chronic intestinal disease, inflammatory bowel disease, predisposition to bowel obstruction and malabsorption syndromes [196]. Moreover, high dosages of acarbose can occasionally increase liver enzyme concentrations [183].

Adverse effects

α-Glucosidase inhibitors have a good safety record, but their application has been limited by gastrointestinal side effects, which represent the main problem, including flatulence, abdominal bloating and discomfort and sometimes diarrhea. They do not cause weight gain or frank hypoglycemia [154].

4. Novel treatment for diabetes mellitus

4.1. Gliptins

Briefly, incretin hormones, glucose-dependent insulinotropic polypeptide (GIP) and glucagon-like peptide 1 (GLP-1), are secreted from the intestine in response to meal digestion; one of their key actions is to increase glucose-induced insulin secretion by the pancreatic islet β-cells, thereby reducing prandial glucose excursions [154]. Moreover, GLP-1 also suppresses glucagon secretion from the islet α-cells and, in preclinical models, proliferation and neogenesis of the β-cell and prevention of β-cell apoptosis has been observed. GLP-1 also delays gastric emptying and suppresses food intake and appetite [197].

It was noted in the 1980s that the incretin effect is reduced in T2DM. However, the peptides can't be administrated straightforward, because they are rapidly degraded by the enzyme, dipeptidyl peptidase-4 (DPP-4). Alternatively gliptins, DPP-4 inhibitors, such as sitagliptin, vildagliptin and more recently saxagliptin, were introduced to enhance incretin levels [154].

Mode of action

Gliptins inhibit the aminopeptidase activity of DPP-4, an enzyme found free and in epithelial cells in most tissues, especially in the intestinal mucosa, which cleaves the N-terminal of the incretins GLP-1 and GIP [198]. Raised endogenous incretin concentrations enhance nutrient-induced insulin secretion, decreasing postprandial hyperglycemia.

Pharmacokinetics

Sitagliptin and vildagliptin are each highly bioavailable, rapidly absorbed and show relatively low plasma protein binding [199]. Most of their doses are eliminated unchanged in the urine, so they are contraindicated in patients with renal impairment or may require dose adjustment [200].

Indications

Gliptins are not licensed to be used as monotherapy in T2DM. Currently, as newly available agents, gliptins tend to be preferred as add-on therapy in patients inadequately controlled by metformin or TZDs. Lack of weight gain makes gliptins suitable for overweight and obese patients [154].

Adverse effects

As there are many natural substrates for DPP-4; including neuropeptide Y, bradykinin, gastrin releasing polypeptide, substance P, insulin-like growth factor I and several chemokines such as monocyte chemotactic protein-1, gliptins have the potential to influence the hunger-satiety system, gastrointestinal motility, growth, vascular reactivity and immune mechanisms [201].

4.2. GLP-1 receptor agonists

As GLP-1 shows important functions in glycemic control, GLP-1 mimetics have been developed. They are designed to be DPP-4 resistant to prolong their plasma half-life. GLP-1 receptor agonists, taken subcutaneously, improve glucose metabolism; mainly by increasing insulin secretion, inhibiting glucagon secretion and delaying gastric emptying[197]. This delay in gastric emptying decreases caloric intake, promoting weight loss. It is unknown whether GLP-1 receptor agonists can delay the progression of T2DM or not. At present, two GLP-1 receptor agonists, exenatide and liraglutide are approved for the treatment of diabetes [202]. Exenatide, a synthetic exendin-4, has shorter half-life than liraglutide, which is a once daily human GLP-1 analog [203]. They both produce a reduction in glucose concentrations, predominately affecting postprandial glycemic excursion, with only modest effects on fasting blood glucose and low risk of hypoglycemia [204].

Adverse effects

The main side effects, as nausea and vomiting, are dose dependent[205]. About 40-50% of treated subjects develop antibodies to exenatide. Exenatide is not recommended for patients with severe kidney failure because it is predominantly eliminated by glomerular filtration [206].

Future GLP-1 receptor agonists, now in phase 3 clinical development

Albiglutide is a long-acting GLP-1 receptor agonist, developed by genetic fusion of a DPP-4 resistant GLP-1 dimer to recombinant human albumin[207]. Despite the large size of the molecule, albiglutide inhibits gastric emptying and appetite, although its anorectic effect may be weaker than that of native GLP-1 because of an impaired blood brain barrier permeability [208].

Taspoglutide is a modified human GLP-1 receptor agonist, taken once weekly [209].

Lixisenatide is a novel modified exendin-4 molecule [210].

4.3. Amylin and amylin analogs

Amylin is a 37 amino acid peptide co-secreted with insulin. It delays gastric emptying, suppresses postprandial glucagon secretion and increases satiety [211]. Human amylin has an inherent tendency to self-aggregate, forming fibrils and to adhere to surfaces. Thus, pramlintide has been developed as an amylin analog with some amino acid replacement. Pramlintide was approved by the FDA in 2005 for use, subcutaneously, in insulin treated subjects with either T1DM or T2DM. Long-term clinical trials have shown quite promising results that the use of pramlintide as an adjunct to insulin minimizes postprandial glucose excursions and reduces both HbA_{1C} and body weight when compared to placebo [212]. It is primarily eliminated by the kidneys [213].

Side effects

The most common side effects are gastrointestinal, often nausea and vomiting but these are generally transient. Hypoglycemia can also occur. However, when the dose is titrated, especially with a reduction in insulin dose, both side effects have been reduced significantly [214].

4.4. Rimonabant

Rimonabant is the first agent of the class of drugs that act on the novel endocannabinoid system (ECS). The ECS is a novel physiological neuroendocrine system that plays a key role in appetite and metabolism, both in brain and adipose tissue. Animal studies have shown that blocking the ECS leads to weight loss and improved insulin sensitivity. Due to this effect, agents that block receptors (CB1 and CB2) in this system have been developed for the management of human obesity. By blocking CB1 receptors in the brain, rimonabant has been shown to reduce weight by suppressing appetite and by modifying glucose and fat metabolism. In the adipose tissue, the drug increases concentrations of adiponectin improving insulin sensitivity [215].

The most common side effects were nausea, vomiting, diarrhea, dizziness, anxiety, depression and suicidal thoughts [216, 217]. These mental disorders result in its withdrawal from the market in 2008 [217].

5. New Experimental Agents

Many potential drugs are currently in investigation. They are undergoing phase I/II studies.

- PPARα/γ ligands (muraglitazar and tesaglitazar - development stopped due to adverse risk profile; aleglitazar - is now under clinical development) [218].
- Sodium-dependent glucose transporter 2 inhibitors (SGLT2 inhibitors) increase urinary glucose excretion [218].
- Fructose 1,6-bisphosphatase inhibitors (FBPase inhibitors) decrease gluconeogenesis in the liver [218].
- Imeglimin is an indirect activator of AMP-kinase acting at the mitochondrial level as an oxidative phosphorylation blocker to inhibit hepatic gluconeogenesis, increase muscle glucose uptake and restore normal insulin secretion. It will be the first of a new class of antidiabetic agents, Glimins, if it is approved. It is in development for use both as monotherapy and in combination with other antidiabetic agents [218].

Treatment strategies for initiation of oral therapy [219]

In patients with newly diagnosed type 2 diabetes;

- Initiate pharmacologic therapy with an oral agent preferably an insulin sensitizer.
  It is recommended to start with metformin, the optimal first line agent, especially in obese patients, or a thiazolidinedione, or a sulfonylurea as monotherapy as long as no contraindication is present. The meglitinides and the α-glucosidase inhibitors are less effective and are less commonly used to initiate therapy. If the blood glucose level is especially high (>280-300 mg/dl) and the patient is symptomatic, insulin should be considered as first-line therapy.

- If monotherapy fails to achieve the desired level of glycemic control, a second oral agent should be added. Various combination tablets are available, including Metaglip (glipizide plus metformin) and Glucovance (glyburide plus metformin).

- In diabetic patients in whom glycemic control is not achieved with two oral agents, several options are available. These include; 1) addition of a third oral antidiabetic agent; 2) addition of bedtime insulin to oral agent therapy; if this option is chosen, to avoid hypoglycemia, it is preferred to stop sulfonylurea and continue the insulin sensitizer; 3) switching the patient to a mixed-split insulin regimen with or without an insulin sensitizer.

It is important to note that, ultimately, most patients with type 2 diabetes will require treatment with insulin, either alone or in combination with an oral agent.

B- Insulin

Insulin is a hormone secreted by pancreatic β-cells, affects a wide range of physiological processes, although it is best known for its important regulatory role in glucose homeostasis. Insulin secretion is increased, in response to elevated plasma glucose, stimulating glucose uptake and glycogen synthesis and inhibiting glycogenolysis and gluconeogenesis, thus maintaining normoglycemia. In addition to these well-established short-term actions, insulin exerts a number of other important metabolic effects, as it regulates the expression of genes involved in amino acid uptake, lipid metabolism in muscle and adipose tissue and in cell growth, development and survival [220].

With the introduction of several new insulins since 1996, insulin therapy became the treatment of type 1 diabetes and, under certain conditions, for type 2 diabetic patients. Insulin therapies are now able to more closely mimic physiologic insulin secretion and thus, achieve better glycemic control in patients with diabetes [221].

In 1955, insulin was the first protein to be fully sequenced. The insulin molecule consists of 51 amino acids arranged in two chains, an A chain (21 amino acids) and B chain (30 amino acids), that are linked by two disulfide bonds. Proinsulin is the insulin precursor that is first processed in the golgi apparatus of the β-cell and then packaged into granules. Proinsulin, a single-chain 86 amino acid peptide, shown in Figure (12), is cleaved into insulin and C-peptide (a connecting peptide); both are secreted in equimolar portions from the β-cell upon stimulation from glucose and other insulin secretagogues. Although proinsulin may have some mild hypoglycemic action, C-peptide has no known physiologic function [222].

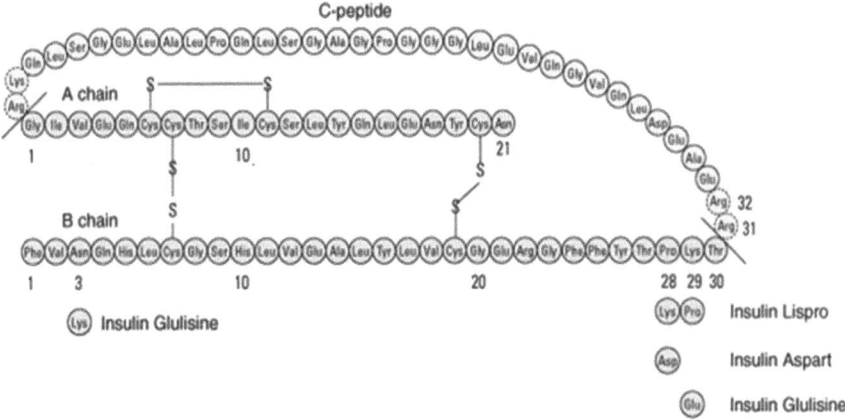

Figure (12): Structure of human proinsulin and some commercially available insulin analogs. Insulin is shown as the shaded peptide chains, A and B. differences in the A and B chains and amino acid modifications for insulin aspart, lispro and glulisine are noted [222].

In general, insulin should be initiated in patients with type 2 diabetes under the following circumstances [223]:

- Symptomatic diabetes (thirst, weight loss, visual impairment or severe hyperglycemia; i.e. fasting plasma glucose > 250 mg/dl)
- Advanced renal or hepatic disease
- Intolerance or contraindications to oral agents or increased risk of a major side effect, such as lactic acidosis with metformin treatment
- Intercurrent events that require hospitalization, such as myocardial infarction, cardiovascular accidents, cerebrovascular accidents, acute illness or surgery
- Hypoperfusion states, such as sepsis or hypotension

- Triglyceride level higher than 700 mg/dl, especially in patients with coronary artery disease, as hypertriglyceridemia worsens insulin resistance and cardiovascular diseases
- Corticosteroid therapy
- Pregnancy
- Ketoacidosis or hyperosmolar states
- Inability to control blood glucose level or reduce HbA_{1C} less than 7% after using combination oral hypoglycemic agents for 4 months or longer
- Latent autoimmune diabetes in adults (LADA); misdiagnosed as type 2 diabetes mellitus

Insulin secretion

Insulin is released from pancreatic β-cells at a low basal rate and at a much higher stimulated rate in response to a variety of stimuli, especially glucose, Figure (13). Other stimulants, such as other sugars (e.g. mannose), certain amino acids (e.g. leucine, arginine), fatty acids, amylin and hormones such as glucagon-like polypeptide-1, are recognized [222].

When evoked by glucose, insulin secretion is biphasic; the first phase reaches a peak after 1 to 2 minutes and is short-lived for 10 minutes, which suppresses hepatic glucose production and facilitates the second phase, which has a delayed onset but a longer duration, lasts two hours and covers mealtime carbohydrates. Between meals, a low continuous insulin level, called basal insulin, serves the ongoing metabolic needs. In type 2 diabetes, first phase release is absent and second phase release is delayed and inadequate [224].

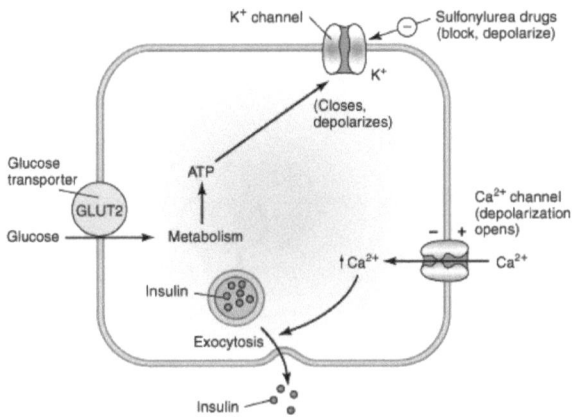

Figure (13): Model of control of insulin release from the pancreatic β-cell by glucose and by sulfonylurea drugs [222].

The insulin receptor

The full insulin receptor consists of two covalently linked heterodimers, each containing an α-subunit, which is entirely extracellular and constitutes the recognition site, and a β-subunit that spans the membrane and contains a tyrosine kinase. The binding of an insulin molecule to the α-subunits at the outside surface of the cell activates the receptor and through a conformational change brings the catalytic loops of the opposing cytoplasmic β-subunits into closer proximity. This facilitates mutual phosphorylation of tyrosine residues on the β-subunits and activates tyrosine kinase directed at cytoplasmic proteins [222]. This is illustrated in Figure (14).

After tyrosine phosphorylation at several critical sites, the IRS molecules bind to and activate other kinases, most significantly phosphatidylinositol-3-kinase, which produce further phosphorylations to adaptor proteins. This network of phosphorylations within the cell represents insulin's second message and results in multiple effects. These include translocation of glucose transporters to the cell membrane with a resultant increase in glucose uptake; increased glycogen synthase activity and increased glycogen formation; multiple effects on protein synthesis and lipogenesis; and activation of transcription factors that enhance DNA synthesis and cell growth and division. Aberrant serine phosphorylation of the insulin receptor β-subunits or IRS molecules may result in insulin resistance and functional receptor down-regulation [222].

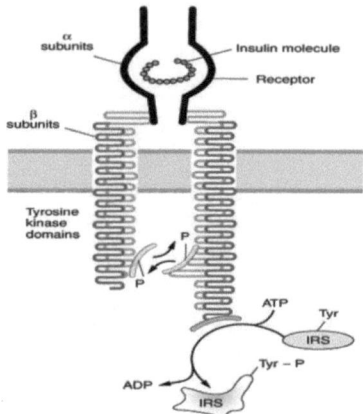

Figure (14): Schematic diagram of the insulin receptor heterodimer in the activated state[222].

Like any receptor, insulin receptors are subjected to up-regulation and increase in responsiveness to insulin in low insulin concentrations, while subjected to down-regulation and decrease in responsiveness to insulin in high insulin concentrations.

Insulin actions on carbohydrate, fat and protein metabolism

Insulin influences glucose metabolism in most tissues, especially the liver, where it inhibits glycogenolysis and gluconeogenesis, decreasing hepatic glucose output and stimulates glycogen synthesis, increasing hepatic glycogen stores. In muscle, unlike liver, uptake of glucose is slow and is the rate-limiting step in carbohydrate metabolism. The main effects of insulin in muscles are to increase facilitated transport of glucose via GLUT4 and to stimulate glycogen synthesis and glycolysis [225].

Insulin increases glucose uptake by GLUT4 in adipose tissue as in muscle, enhancing glucose metabolism. Moreover, it increases synthesis of fatty acid and triglyceride in adipose tissue and in liver. It inhibits lipolysis, partly via dephosphorylation (and hence inactivation) of lipases [225].

Insulin stimulates uptake of amino acids into muscle and increases protein synthesis. It also decreases protein catabolism and inhibits oxidation of amino acids in the liver [225].

In addition, insulin increases the permeability of many cells to potassium, magnesium and phosphate ions. The effect on potassium is clinically important. Insulin activates sodium-potassium ATPases in many cells, causing a flux of potassium into cells. Under certain circumstances, injection of insulin can kill patients because of its ability to acutely suppress plasma potassium concentrations [225].

Insulin pharmacokinetics

Endogenous insulin passes through the portal vein to the liver, where extensive metabolism occurs. The rest enters the systemic circulation, where its concentration is only about 15% of that entering the liver in fasting state. In contrast, when insulin is injected subcutaneously, intramuscularly or intravenously, it enters the systemic circulation and then distributes to all tissues (the liver and other peripheral organs) in the same concentration. Therefore, during insulin treatment, liver is relatively hypoinsulinized and the peripheral tissues are relatively hyperinsulinized. Intravenous administration (continuous or pulse) is not practical but permits much more physiological insulin profiles. Other routes of insulin delivery have been proposed, including the intraperitoneal route (which allows insulin to enter, at least in part, the portal vein, similarly to the endogenously secreted insulin), transdermal insulin patches (yielded disappointing results) and rectal suppositories (unable to induce a physiological profile of insulinemia) [226].

Research into oral administration of insulin has been ongoing for several years. Oral delivery of insulin is restricted mainly due to its susceptibility to denaturation and proteolysis, as well as its inability to traverse across biological barriers [227, 228]. Various approaches have been adopted to overcome the inherent barriers for oral insulin, including chemical modification of insulin and co-administration of adjuvants; either in the form of absorption enhancers or protease inhibitors. Among the promising effective approaches towards developing oral insulin delivery systems is the use of polymeric nanoparticles [228]. The insulin loaded nanoparticles coated with the mucoadhesive chitosan, an intestinal permeation enhancer, may prolong their residency in the gut, protect them from gastric enzymes and enhance permeability by disrupting tight junctions between gut epithelial cells, thus allowing the drug to reach its ultimate bloodstream destination [227, 228].

Inhaled insulin is a powder form of recombinant DNA (rDNA) human insulin that is administered through an inhaler device. Insulin is readily absorbed into the bloodstream through alveolar walls, but the challenge has been to create particles that are small enough to pass through the bronchial tree without being trapped and still enter the alveoli in sufficient amounts to have a clinical effect [222].

Insulin preparations

Effects of insulin therapy and its mechanism of action are the same as normal insulin. Insulin for clinical use was once either porcine or bovine, but is now almost entirely human (made by recombinant DNA technology). Porcine and bovine insulins differ from human insulin in their amino acid sequence and are liable to elicit an immune response, a problem that is avoided by the use of recombinant human insulin. Commercial insulin preparations are highly purified and differ in a number of ways, such as differences in the recombinant DNA production techniques, amino acid sequence, concentration, solubility and the time of onset and duration of their biologic action [222].

(1) Ultra-short-acting, with very fast onset and short duration; taken before meals;
e.g. insulin lispro, insulin aspart and insulin glulisine [229].

(2) Short-acting, with rapid onset of action; Regular insulin, which is a soluble crystalline zinc insulin. Its effect appears within 30 minutes and peaks between 2 and 3 hours after subcutaneous injection and generally lasts 5-8 hours [222].

(3) Intermediate-acting; NPH (Neutral Protamine Hagedorn, or Isophane), its absorption and the onset of action are delayed by combining appropriate amounts of insulin and protamine, so that neither is present in an uncomplexed form "isophane" [222]. Another intermediate acting

analogue is "Lente insulin", which is a mixture of 3:7 semilente and ultralente. They have an onset of approximately 1-2 hours and duration of 18-24 hours [219].

(4) Long-acting, with slow onset of action; Ultralente insulin has an onset of action 4-6 hours, a peak effect 16-18 hours after injection and a duration of action up to 36 hours [219].

(5) Ultra-long-acting insulin analog; Insulin Glargine (Lantus®) is a soluble, "peakless" (i.e. having a broad plasma concentration plateau). This product was designed to provide reproducible and convenient insulin replacement [222], through providing a constant basal insulin supply that mimics the physiological insulin secretion [230].

Insulin detemir is a most recently developed long-acting insulin analog, designed to prolong its availability by increasing both self-aggregation in subcutaneous tissue and reversible albumin binding [231].

Insulin degludec is a novel insulin analog in clinical development that forms soluble multihexamer assemblies after subcutaneous injection, resulting in an ultra-long duration of action [232].

Uses of insulin [225]

- For treatment of type 1 and type 2 diabetes mellitus, which are the primary indications for insulin therapy
- For hyperkalemia, as insulin promotes the passage of potassium simultaneously with glucose into cells
- In anterior pituitary function test (the insulin stress test)

Adverse effects of insulin

1- Hypoglycemia is the most frequent and feared complication of insulin treatment, with potentially serious sequelae [233]. Poor timing of meals, exercise and insulin treatment can lead to hypoglycemia, which may lead to coma, convulsions and even death, mainly due to glucose deprivation in brain [234].

2- Weight gain is also among insulin adverse effects. Improved glycemic control decreases glucosuria; thereby decreasing the loss of calories through the urine and the direct lipogenic effects of insulin on adipose tissue, both contribute to weight gain [233].

3- Insulin lipodystrophy (lipoatrophy or lipohypertrophy) can occur after repeated administration of insulin at the same injection site; however, these are rare with purified human insulin. Lipoatrophy might be the result of a repeated mechanical trauma. In addition, insulin impurities can stimulate immune factors, which lead to local release of lipolytic substances [235]. On the other hand, lipohypertrophy is due to a possible growth factor effect of insulin on cellular elements of subcutaneous tissue [226]. Both may alter the absorption rate of insulin, thus possibly affecting the metabolic control.

4- Local allergy or generalized allergy, ranging from a simple urticaria to more severe reactions, such as anaphylaxis, may occur [226].

Management of diabetic dyslipidemia: [236]

In type 2 diabetes mellitus, an increased prevalence of lipid abnormalities contributes to the accelerated atherosclerosis, thus aggressive screening of these abnormalities are essential. A fasting lipid profile is recommended at the initial evaluation and at least annually for adults with T2DM because frequent changes in glycemic control may affect lipoprotein levels. In adults with low risk lipid values, repeated assessments can be done every 2 years.

The target lipid profile is to reduce LDL to <100 mg/dl or to < 70 mg/dl in high risk patients and triglycerides to < 150 mg/dl as well as increase HDL to > 40 mg/dl for men and to > 50 mg/dl for women. Non-HDL-C can be targeted in patients with triglycerides ≥ 200 mg/dl, its goal is ≤ 130 mg/dl.

- Achieve optimal glycemic control and maximal adherence to therapeutic and lifestyle changes.
- Lowering LDL-C to the target level is the primary goal of therapy. For patients, more than 40 years of age, statin therapy, HMG-CoA reductase inhibitors, is recommended to achieve a LDL-C reduction of 30-40%, regardless of baseline LDL levels. Statins are the most effective LDL-C lowering medication with an excellent safety

profile. They are effective in lowering cardiovascular events independent of baseline LDL, pre-existing vascular disease, type or duration of diabetes or adequacy of glycemic control. In patients who do not achieve LDL cholesterol targets, bile acid sequestrants and cholesterol absorption inhibitors can be used for further reduction of LDL-C levels.

- Fibrates, particularly fenofibrate and niacin, are primarily used to lower triglycerides and raise HDL-C levels, to achieve target levels. In addition, they can reduce LDL-C levels as well.
- Combination therapy using statins and fibrates or niacin may be necessary to achieve lipid targets in some patients.
- In the presence of dyslipidemia, characterized predominantly by severely elevated triglycerides (>500 mg/dl), it should be aggressively managed, as it is considered a risk factor for pancreatitis [51]. A fibrate is recommended, but additional therapy with niacin and omega-3-fatty acid may be required.

Management of diabetic complications: [236]

- Concerning cardiovascular diseases, low dose aspirin and an angiotensin converting enzyme inhibitors (ACEI) or an angiotensin receptor blocker (ARB) are recommended to diabetic patients with hypertension, as they decrease myocardial infarction risk and can confer unique protective effects.
- Guidelines advocate for the use of ACEI or ARBs for microalbuminuria, even in non-hypertensive patients, because of their ability to slow its progression to clinical proteinuria, as well as the latter to end stage renal failure (ESRF). In further progression in renal insufficiency, the essential approaches are managing the secondary complications as anemia and hyperparathyroidism, as well as managing protein intake, hyperphosphatemia hyperkalemia and the overall nutrition. However, in ESRF, dialysis and transplantation are the available managing options.
- Panretinal photocoagulation is considered the treatment of choice for patients with proliferative retinopathy, which is used to stop

neovascularization before recurrent hemorrhages into the vitreous, causing irreparable damage.
- Infected foot ulcers usually require intravenous antibiotics, bed rest with foot elevation and surgical debridement. In addition, reducing plantar pressure, using specialized footwear, accelerates healing.
- Intensive control of hyperglycemia and hypertension, as well as control the pain if presents, represent the primary tools in the prevention and management of neuropathy. Tricyclic antidepressants, antiseziure medications with analgesics may be helpful in some patients with painful neuropathy. Physical therapy is often helpful.
- Metoclopramide and domperidone are effective in gastroparesis.
- Patients with orthostatic hypotension can benefit from non-pharmacological and pharmacological interventions (midodrine and caffeine), used to treat this condition.

AIM OF THE WORK

The aim of present study is to evaluate the possible effects of oral treatment with the antidiabetic drug metformin and the antioxidant amino acid L-cysteine, when used alone or in combination, in streptozotocin experimentally-induced diabetic rats. Moreover, it was aimed to shed a light on the glycemic control, lipid profile, inflammatory markers and hepatic tissue oxidative stress changes occurring in streptozotocin experimentally-induced diabetic rats.

MATERIALS AND METHODS

1-Experimental animals

In the present study, 50 adult male albino Wistar rats 3-4 months old, weighing between 170-200 gm, were used. The rats were obtained from the animal house of the Medical Research Institute, Alexandria University. All rats were kept under observation for at least one week prior to study with free access to food and water for acclimatization. Rats were exposed to alternate cycle of 12 hours light and 12 hours darkness. They were put in pairs in transparent cages under good sanitary conditions and normal humidity. All procedures were performed in accordance with regulations of the National Research Council's guide for the care and use of laboratory animals.

2-Induction of type 2 diabetes mellitus in rats

To develop a rat model of experimentally-induced type 2 diabetes mellitus, which resembles that occurring in human population, overnight fasting rats were injected intravenously with low dose streptozotocin (15 mg/kg) after high fat diet for two months. The solution was freshly prepared and was injected via the caudal vein. Diabetes was confirmed 3 days later by blood glucose level 200-300 mg/dl for 2 consecutive days in fed animals.

3-Drugs and doses

1- Streptozotocin (Sigma Aldrich Co-USA), dissolved in 0.1M citrate buffer pH 4.5 and injected intravenously through the caudal vein in a dose 15 mg/kg [237].

2- Metformin HCl (Pharco Pharmaceuticals, Alexandria, Egypt), dissolved in distilled water and given by oral gavage to the rats in a dose 300 mg/kg/day [238].

3- L-cysteine (Sigma Co Ltd-England) dissolved in distilled water and given by oral gavage to the rats in a dose 300 mg/kg/day [239].

4- Experimental design

In the present study, rats were divided into five groups, 10 rats each. In all groups, except group V, rats were kept on a high fat diet (30% fat) for 2 months, after which they were rendered diabetic by streptozotocin injection intravenously. After induction of diabetes, drug treatment was carried out for 2 weeks as follows:

Group I: Received distilled water orally and served as untreated diabetic control.

Group II: Treated orally with 300mg/kg/day metformin HCl dissolved in distilled water.

Group III: Treated orally with 300mg/kg/day L-cysteine dissolved in distilled water.

Group IV: Treated orally with both metformin HCl (300mg/kg/day) and L-cysteine (300mg/kg/day) in distilled water.

Group V: Fed conventional rat chow and served as normal non-diabetic control.

After 2 weeks of treatment, overnight fasting rats were sacrificed by decapitation. Blood was collected and serum was separated for the determination of the following biochemical metabolic parameters:

1- Fasting glucose level [240].
2- Insulin [241].
3- Triglycerides [242].
4- Total cholesterol [243].
5- HDL [244].
6- LDL [245].
7- Free fatty acids [246].
8- Monocyte chemoattractant protein-1 (MCP-1) [247, 248].
9- C-reactive protein [249].
10- Nitric oxide [250].

Immediately after collection of blood, livers were excised, washed with ice-cold saline and preserved for the assessment of:

1- Malondialdehyde level [251].
2- Reduced glutathione [252].
3- Protein content [253].

I- Biochemical metabolic parameters

1- Determination of fasting serum glucose levels [240]

Reaction principle

According to Trinder's method, serum glucose was determined after enzymatic oxidation in the presence of glucose oxidase. The formed hydrogen peroxide reacts under catalysis of peroxidase, with phenol and 4-aminophenazone to a red-violet quinoneimine as an indicator.

$$\text{Glucose} + O_2 + H_2O \xrightarrow{\text{Glucose Oxidase}} \text{Gluconic acid} + 4H_2O_2$$

$$2H_2O_2 + \text{4-aminophenazone} + \text{phenol} \xrightarrow{\text{Peroxidase}} \text{Quinoneimine} + 4H_2O$$

Reagents

1- Enzyme reagent

Phosphate buffer (pH 7.5)	0.1 mmol/L
4-aminophenazone	0.25 mmol/L
Phenol	0.75 mmol/L
Glucose oxidase	>15 KU/L
Peroxidase	>1.5 KU/L
Mutarotase	>2.0 KU/L

2- Standard   100 mg/dl (5.55 mmol/L)

Method

In a spectrophotometer cuvette, the following reagents were pipetted

- 20 µl sample
- 2000 µl enzyme reagent

The contents were mixed and then incubated for 5 minutes at 37°C. The absorbance was read at 500 nm within 60 minutes against a blank containing only 2000 µl of the enzyme reagent. The same procedure was repeated using 20 µl of the standard instead of the sample.

Calculation

Concentration of fasting serum glucose (mg/dl) = $\dfrac{\text{Absorbance of sample}}{\text{Absorbance of standard}} \times 100$

2- Determination of fasting serum insulin [241]

Serum insulin was determined according to Bank's method by an in-vitro enzyme linked immunosorbent assay using ALPCO® insulin (rat) ELISA kit.

Principle of the assay:

This assay is a sandwich type immunoassay based on the immobilization of monoclonal antibodies specific for insulin as the solid phase. Insulin molecules present in the sample become bound to the wells by the immobilized antibody then reacts with a horseradish peroxidase enzyme labeled monoclonal antibody (conjugate), resulting in insulin molecules being sandwiched between the solid phase and the conjugate. On using 3,3',5,5' tetramethylbenzidine (TMB) as a substrate, a blue color is formed which then changes to yellow color after addition of a stop solution. The intensity of the color generated is directly proportional to the amount of insulin in the sample.

Reagents

- 96 well insulin microplate, coated with mouse monoclonal anti-insulin
- Zero standard (0 ng/ml)
- Standards (A → E) (0.15, 0.4, 1, 3, 5.5 ng/ml)
- Mammalian insulin high and low controls, reconstituted each in 0.6 ml distilled water.
- Conjugate stock 11X (HRP labeled monoclonal anti-insulin antibody), diluted with 10 parts conjugate buffer
- Wash buffer concentrate 21X, diluted with 20 parts distilled water.
- TMB substrate (3,3',5,5' tetramethylbenzidine)
- Stop solution (0.3 M HCl)

Method

All reagents, samples and microplate strips were brought to room temperature.

1. 10 µl of each standard, reconstituted control, or sample were pipetted into its respective well.
2. 75 µl of working strength conjugate was pipetted into each well.
3. The microplate was incubated for 2 hours at room temperature (18-25°C), on a horizontal microplate shaker (at 700-900 rpm).
4. After incubation, the microplate was washed 6 times with working strength wash buffer then 100 µl of TMB substrate was pipetted into each well.
5. The microplate was again incubated with shaking (at 700-900 rpm) for 15 minutes at room temperature (18-25°C).
6. 100 µl of stop solution was pipetted into each well with gentle shaking to stop the reaction.
7. The absorbance was read at 450 nm within 30 minutes following the addition of stop solution.

Calculation

The concentration of serum insulin in the samples was determined in ng/ml from a calibration curve, which was constructed from the standards. The zero standard was used as a blank with its average value subtracted from each well.

The calibration curve of insulin is illustrated in Figure (15).

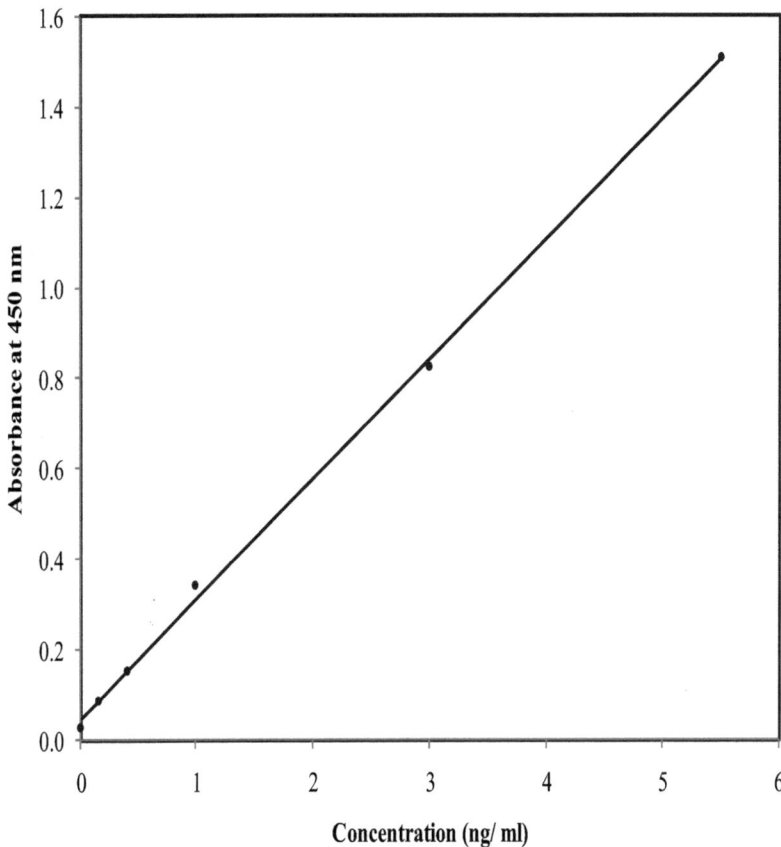

Figure (15): Standard curve of insulin

3- Determination of serum triglycerides [242]

Reaction principle

The determination of serum triglycerides was carried out according to Rifai's method. Triglycerides were determined after enzymatic hydrolysis with lipases by a colorimetric method. The indicator is a quinoneimine derivative formed from hydrogen peroxide, 4-aminoantipyrine and p-chlorophenol under the catalytic influence of peroxidase.

$$\text{Triglycerides} + H_2O \xrightarrow{\text{Lipases}} \text{Glycerol} + \text{Fatty acids}$$

$$\text{Glycerol} + ATP \xrightarrow{\text{Glycerol Kinase}} \text{Glycerol-3-phosphate} + ADP$$

$$\text{Glycerol-3-phosphate} + O_2 \xrightarrow{\text{Gycerol-3 P-oxidase}} \text{Dihydroacetone phosphate} + H_2O_2$$

$$2H_2O_2 + \text{4-aminoantipyrine} + \text{p-chlorophenol} \xrightarrow{\text{Peroxidase}} \text{Quinoneimine} + 4 H_2O + HCl$$

Reagents

1- Reagent 1

Pipes buffer	50 mmol/L, pH 7.00
p-Chlorophenol	2.7 mmol/L
Magnesium ions	14.8 mmol/L
ATP	3.15 mmol/L
Potassium ferrocyanide	10 µmol/L
4-aminoantipyrine	0.31 mmol/L
Lipoprotein lipases	≥2000 U/L
Glycerol kinase	≥500 U/L
Glycerol-3-phosphate oxidase	≥4000 U/L
Peroxidase	≥500 U/L

2- Reagent 2 (Standard): Glycerol (triglycerides equivalent); 200 mg/dl (2.28 mmol/L).

Method

In a spectrophotometer cuvette, the following reagents were pipetted

- 3 µl sample
- 300 µl reagent 1

The contents were mixed then incubated for 10 minutes at 37°C. The absorbance was read at 500 nm against a blank containing 300 µl of reagent 1 with 3 µl distilled water. The same procedure was repeated using 3 µl of the standard instead of the sample.

Calculation

Concentration of serum triglycerides (mg/dl) = $\dfrac{\text{Absorbance of sample}}{\text{Absorbance of standard}}$ X 200

4-Determination of serum total cholesterol [243]

Reaction principle

Serum total cholesterol was determined according to Allian's method. After enzymatic hydrolysis and oxidation of cholesterol, the reaction product, hydrogen peroxide forms a red violet indicator (quinoneimine) with 4-aminoantipyrine and phenol under the catalytic action of peroxidase.

$$\text{Cholesterol ester} + H_2O \xrightarrow{\text{Cholesterol Esterase}} \text{Cholesterol} + \text{fatty acids}$$

$$\text{Cholesterol} + O_2 \xrightarrow{\text{Cholesterol Oxidase}} \text{3-Cholesterolone} + H_2O_2$$

$$2H_2O_2 + \text{4-aminoantipyrine} + \text{phenol} \xrightarrow{\text{Peroxidase}} \text{Quinoneimine} + 4H_2O$$

Reagents

Reagent 1 (Color reagent):

- Good's buffer (pH 6.7)	50 mmol/L
- Phenol	5 mmol/L
- 4-aminoantipyrine	0.3 mmol/L
- Cholesterol esterase	≥200 U/L

- Cholesterol oxidase ≥50 U/L
- Peroxidase ≥3000 U/L

Reagent 2 (Standard): 200 mg/dl (5.2 mmol/L)

Method

In a spectrophotometer cuvette, the following reagents were pipetted

- 10 µl sample
- 1000 µl color reagent (R_1)

The contents were mixed then incubated for 10 minutes at 37°C. The absorbance was read at 500 nm within 60 minutes against a blank containing 1000 µl of color reagent (R_1) with 10 µl distilled water. The same procedure was repeated using 10 µl of the standard (R_2) instead of the sample.

Calculation

$$\text{Concentration of serum total cholesterol (mg/dl)} = \frac{\text{Absorbance of sample}}{\text{Absorbance of standard}} \times 200$$

5-Determination of serum HDL-cholesterol [244]

Reaction principle

The determination of serum HDL-cholesterol was carried out according to Grove's method. Very low-density lipoproteins (VLDL) and low-density lipoproteins (LDL) in the sample are precipitated with phosphotungestate and magnesium ions. The supernatant contains high-density lipoproteins. The HDL-cholesterol is then spectrophotometerically measured by means of the coupled reactions described below:

$$\text{Cholesterol ester} + H_2O \xrightarrow{\text{Cholesterol Esterase}} \text{Cholesterol} + \text{fatty acids}$$

$$\text{Cholesterol} + \tfrac{1}{2} O_2 + H_2O \xrightarrow{\text{Cholesterol Oxidase}} \text{Cholestenone} + H_2O_2$$

$$2H_2O_2 + \text{4-aminoantipyrine} + \text{phenol} \xrightarrow{\text{Peroxidase}} \text{Quinoneimine} + 4H_2O$$

Reagents

Reagent A

    Phosphotungestate   0.4 mmol/L

    Magnesium chloride   20 mmol/L

Reagent B (Color reagent)

HDL-cholesterol standard   15 mg/dl

Method

1- A mixture of 0.2 ml sample and 0.5 ml reagent A was left to stand for 10 minutes at room temperature and then centrifuged at a minimum of 4000 rpm for 10 minutes. The supernatant was then carefully collected.

2- 0.1 ml of the clear supernatant was pipetted into a spectrophotometer cuvette, followed by the addition of 1 ml of color reagent B and incubated for 10 minutes at 37°C.

3- The absorbance was read at 500 nm within 30 minutes against a blank containing 100 µl of distilled water and 1 ml of reagent B. The sample procedure was repeated using 100 µl of the HDL-cholesterol standard instead of the sample.

Calculation

$$\text{Concentration of serum HDL-cholesterol (mg/dl)} = \frac{\text{Absorbance of sample}}{\text{Absorbance of standard}} \times 52.5$$

6-Determination of serum LDL-cholesterol [245]

Reaction principle

Low-density lipoproteins (LDL) were determined according to Friedewald's method. LDL in the sample is precipitated with polyvinyl sulphate. Their concentration is calculated from the difference between the serum total cholesterol and the cholesterol in the supernatant after centrifugation. The cholesterol is spectrophotometerically measured by means of the coupled reaction described below:

Cholesterol esters + H_2O $\xrightarrow{\text{Cholesterol Esterase}}$ Cholesterol + Fatty acids

Cholesterol + ½ O_2 + H_2O $\xrightarrow{\text{Cholesterol Oxidase}}$ Cholestenone + H_2O_2

$2H_2O_2$ + 4-aminoantipyrine + phenol $\xrightarrow{\text{Peroxidase}}$ Quinoneimine + $4H_2O$

Reagents

Reagent A

| Polyvinyl sulphate | 3 gm/L |
| Polyethylene glycol | 3 gm/L |

Reagent B (Color reagent)

Reagent C (Standard):   200 mg/dl (5.2 mmol/L)

Method

1- 0.4 ml of sample and 0.2 ml of reagent A were mixed thoroughly and was left to stand for 14 minutes at room temperature then centrifuged at a minimum of 4000 rpm for 15 minutes.

2- In a spectrophotometer cuvette, 20 µl of the sample supernatant was mixed thoroughly with 1 ml reagent B and then incubated for 10 minutes at 37°C.

3- The absorbance was read at 500 nm against a blank containing 20 µl distilled water instead of sample. The same procedure was repeated using 20 µl of cholesterol standard (reagent C).

Calculation

Cholesterol in supernatant (mg/dl) = Absorbance of sample X 200 X 1.5

The LDL-cholesterol concentration in the sample is calculated as follows:

LDL-cholesterol (mg/dl) = Total cholesterol – cholesterol in the supernatant

7-Determination of serum free fatty acids [246]

Reaction principle

FFAs were determined according to Shimizus's method. FFAs are converted by acyl-CoA synthetase (Acyl CS) into acyl-coenzyme A (acyl-CoA), which reacts with oxygen in the presence of acyl-CoA oxidase (ACOD) to form 2,3-enoyl-coenzyme A (enoyl-CoA). The resulting hydrogen peroxide converts 2,4,4-tribromo-3-hydroxy-benzoic acid (TBHB) and 4-aminoantipyrine to a red dye in the presence of peroxidase.

Free fatty acids + CoA + ATP $\xrightarrow{AcylCS}$ Acyl-CoA + AMP + pyrophosphate

Acyl-CoA + O_2 $\xrightarrow{ACOD}$ Enoyl-CoA + H_2O_2

H_2O_2 + 4-aminoantipyrine + TBHB $\xrightarrow{Peroxidase}$ Red dye + $2H_2O$ + HBr

Reagents

- Reaction mixture A
  - ATP, coenzyme A, acyl-CoA-synthetase, peroxidase, ascorbate oxidase,
    4-aminoantipyrine dissolved in potassium phosphate buffer pH 7.8.
  - Tribromohydroxy-benzoic acid, magnesium chloride and stabilizers.

- Reaction mixture B: Acyl-CoA-oxidase (ACOD) and stabilizers in dilute solution.

- N-ethyl-maleinimide solution with stabilizers.

Method

In a spectrophotometer cuvette, 50 µl of sample and 1 ml of reaction mixture A were mixed, kept at 25°C for approximately 10 minutes, then 0.05 ml of N-ethyl-maleinimide solution was added. The reagents were mixed again, and the absorbance (A_1) was read at wavelength of 546 nm. This was followed by the addition of 50 µl of reaction mixture B and the absorbance (A_2) was read again after 15 minutes.

The same procedure was repeated for the blank, using 0.05 ml of distilled water instead of the sample. The absorbance differences (A_2-A_1) was calculated for both blank and sample.

Calculation

Concentration of serum free fatty acids (mmol/L) = $\dfrac{1.15}{19.3 \times 1 \times 0.05}$ X ΔA = 1.192 X ΔA

Where:

- ΔA = Δ absorbance difference of sample - absorbance difference of blank
- 1.15 = final volume in ml
- 19.3 = absorption coefficient of dyestuff at 546 nm
- 1 = light path in cm
- 0.05 = sample volume

8- Determination of serum monocyte chemoattractant protein-1 [247, 248]

Serum MCP-1 was determined by an in-vitro enzyme-linked immunosorbent assay using RayBio® rat MCP-1 ELISA kit.

Principle of the assay

This assay is based on the immobilization of an antibodies specific for rat MCP-1 as the solid phase. MCP-1 present in the serum sample becomes bound to the wells by the immobilized antibodies then reacts with biotinylated anti-rat MCP-1 antibodies. On adding horseradish peroxidase enzyme (HRP) conjugated streptavidin and 3,3',5,5' tetramethylbenzidine (TMB), a blue color is formed, which then changes to yellow color after addition of a stop solution. The intensity of the color generated is directly proportional to the amount of MCP-1 in the sample.

Reagents

1. 96 well MCP-1 microplate coated with anti-rat MCP-1.
2. Wash buffer concentrate (20X): diluted with 19 parts distilled water.

3. Standards: recombinant rat MCP-1, reconstituted with diluents A to prepare serial dilutions of MCP-1 standards.
4. Assay diluent A: 0.09% sodium azide as preservative and used as a diluent for standard/sample.
5. Assay diluent B (5X): diluted with 4 parts distilled water.
6. Detection biotinylated anti-rat MCP-1 antibodies: reconstituted with 100 µl of 1X assay diluents B and then diluted 65 fold with 1X diluent B.
7. Horseradish peroxidase enzyme (HRP)-conjugated streptavidin: diluted 5000 fold with 1X diluent B.
8. TMB substrate (3,3',5,5' tetramethylbenzidine).
9. Stop solution: 2 M sulfuric acid.

Method:

All reagents and samples were brought to room temperature (18-25°C) before use.

1. 100 µl of each standard and sample were added into appropriate wells. The microplate was covered well and incubated for 2.5 hours at room temperature or overnight at 4°C with gentle shaking.
2. The solution was discarded and washed 4 times with 1X wash solution using an autowasher. After the last wash, any remaining wash buffer was removed.
3. 100 µl of 1x prepared biotinylated antibody was added to each well. The microplate was incubated again for 1 hour at room temperature with gentle shaking.
4. The solution was discarded and the wash was repeated.
5. 100 µl of prepared streptavidin solution was added to each well. The microplate was incubated again for 45 minutes at room temperature with gentle shaking after which the solution was discarded and the wash was repeated.
6. 100 µl of TMB (one-step substrate reagent) was added to each well and the microplate was incubated again for 30 minutes at room temperature in the dark with gentle shaking.
7. 50 µl of stop solution was added to each well and the absorbance was read at 450 nm immediately.

Calculation

The concentration of serum MCP-1 in the samples was determined in pg/ml from a calibration curve, which was constructed from the standards. The zero standard was used as a blank with its average value subtracted from each well.

The calibration curve of MCP-1 is illustrated in Figure (16).

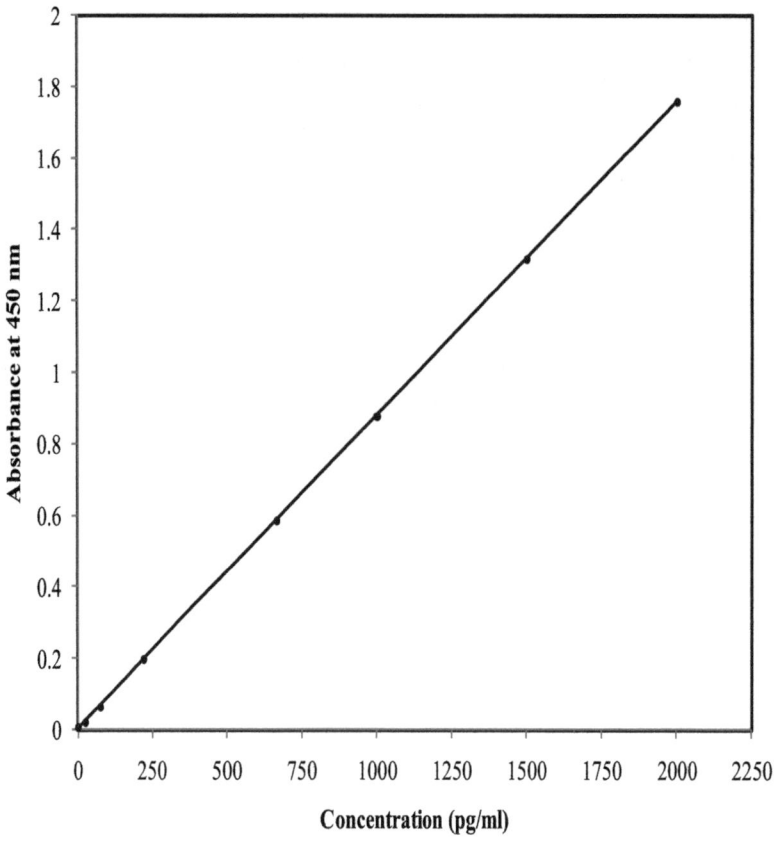

Figure (16): Standard curve of monocyte chemoattractant protein-1 (MCP-1)

9- Determination of serum C-reactive protein [249]

Reaction principle

The serum level of CRP was measured by turbidimetric immunoassay according to Otsuji's method, using an N-Assay TIA CRP-S kit (Nittobo Medical, Tokyo). Serum C-reactive protein causes agglutination of the latex particles coated with anti-rat C-reactive protein. The agglutination of the latex particles is proportional to the CRP concentration and can be measured by turbidimetry.

Reagents

Reagent A: Glycine buffer 0.1 mol/L, sodium azide 0.95 gm/L, pH 8.6

Reagent B: Suspension of the latex particles coated with anti-rat CRP antibodies, sodium azide 0.95 gm/L

Reagent C: CRP standard C-reactive protein 65.6 mg/L

Working reagent: A mixture of reagent A and B

Method

In a spectrophotometer cuvette, the following reagents were pipetted

- 1 ml working reagent
- 7 µl sample

The contents were mixed then the absorbance was read at 540 nm against a blank containing 7 µl distilled water after 10 seconds (A_1) and after 2 minutes (A_2) The same procedure was repeated using 7 µl of the standard (reagent C) instead of the sample.

Calculation

The concentration of serum CRP (mg/L) = $\dfrac{(A_2 - A_1)_{sample}}{(A_2 - A_1)_{standard}} \times 65.6$

10- Determination of serum nitric oxide end products (nitrite NO_2^- and nitrate NO_3^-) [250]

Principle

The nitrite and nitrate concentration was determined by simple Griess reaction. Because the nitric oxide (NO) has a short half-life (2-30 sec), it is preferable to determine nitrite, the stable product of NO, which may be further oxidized to nitrate. So, the Griess reaction was supplemented with the reduction of nitrate to nitrite by NADPH-dependent nitrate reductase.

Reagents

- Nitrate reductase from Aspergillus niger (3 U/ml) in phosphate buffer saline
- 0.32 mM NADPH in 20 mM Tris buffer pH 7.6.
- Methanol: diethyl ether (3:1 v/v)
- 6.5 M HCl.
- 37.5 mM sulphanilic acid.
- 12.5 mM N-(1-naphthyl) ethylenediamine (NED)
- Standard sodium nitrite solution (from 0 to 100 µmol/L)

Procedure

1 -Nitrate reduction and deproteinization

An aliquot of 100 µl of serum was incubated with 50 µl nitrate reductase and 50 µl of NADPH for 30 minutes at room temperature. After the reduction, 100 µl of the mixture was incubated overnight with 900 µl methanol: diethyl ether (3:1 v/v). After the overnight incubation, the sample was centrifuged at 10000 rpm for 10 min at 40°C and the supernatant was used for determination of nitrite.

2 -Nitrite determination

Aliquots of 600 µl of the deproteinized sample, 150 µl of 6.5 M HCl, and 150 µl of 37.5 mM sulphanilic acid were added to a centrifuge tube and then incubated at 40°C for 30 min. After incubation, 150 µl of 12.5 mM NED was added and the sample was centrifuged at 10000 rpm for 10 min at 40°C. The absorbance of the clear supernatant was measured at 540 nm.

Calculation

The concentration of NO in the samples was determined in nmol/ml from a calibration curve, which was constructed by preparing serial concentrations of sodium nitrite, Figure (17).

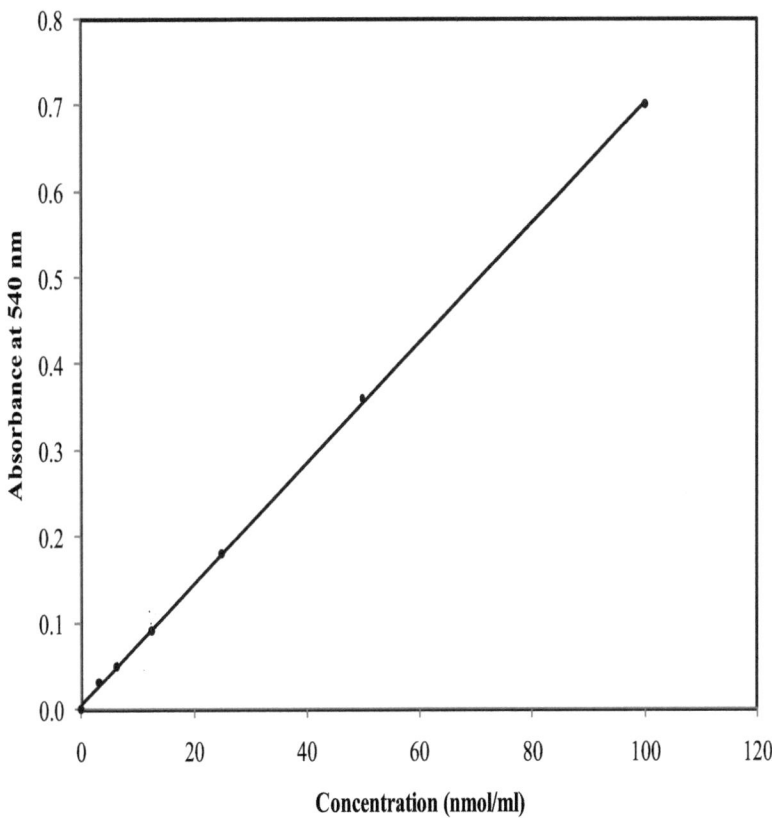

Figure (17): Standard curve of nitric oxide

II- Oxidative stress parameters

1-Determination of hepatic malondialdehyde (MDA) by thiobarbituric acid reaction [251]

Reaction principle

Hepatic malondialdehyde was determined by the thiobarbituric acid (TBA) method, which was described by Ohkawa, for the assay of lipid peroxides in various animal studies. This thiobarbituric acid (TBA) test is most frequently used as an index of lipid peroxidation. It depends on the fact that, when polyunsaturated fatty acids (PUFAs) or esters containing 3 or more double bonds undergo auto-oxidation, a secondary product of lipid peroxidation, which is referred to as malondialdehyde is produced. In this assay, one molecule of malondialdehyde, the most abundant aldehyde product of lipid peroxidation, reacts with two molecules of thiobarbituric acid (TBA) at pH 3.5 to yield a pink chromagen that can be detected spectrophotometerically at 532 nm.

Reagents

- 1.15% potassium chloride.
- 0.8% thiobarbituric acid (TBA) in distilled water
- 8.1% sodium dodecyl sulphate (SDS) in distilled water
- 20% acetic acid (pH 3.5 was adjusted with 1 N NaOH)
- N-butanol
- 1,1, 3,3-tetramethoxypropane (TMP)

Method

1- A small part of the liver was cut, weighed and homogenized in 9 volumes of 1.15% KCl to prepare 10% homogenate (w/v).

2- An aliquot of 0.1 ml liver homogenate was added to 0.2 ml of SDS. This was followed by the addition of 1.5 ml of acetic acid and 1.5 ml of aqueous solution of TBA. This mixture was finally made up to 4 ml with distilled water, vortexed and then heated in a water bath at 95 °C for 60 minutes.

3- After cooling to room temperature, 1 ml of distilled water and 5 ml of n-butanol were added followed by the vigorous shaking. After centrifugation at 4000 rpm for 10 minutes, the absorbance of the organic layer was read at 532 nm using Jenway 6305 spectrophotometer against a blank containing 0.1 ml distilled water instead of the sample and treated exactly like the sample.

Calculation

The level of MDA in the samples in nmol/gm tissue was determined from a standard curve made by preparing serial dilutions of 1,1,3,3-tetramethoxypropane (TMP) (Sigma Chemical Co-USA) in 97% ethanol and treating them like the samples.

The standard curve of MDA is shown in Figure (18).

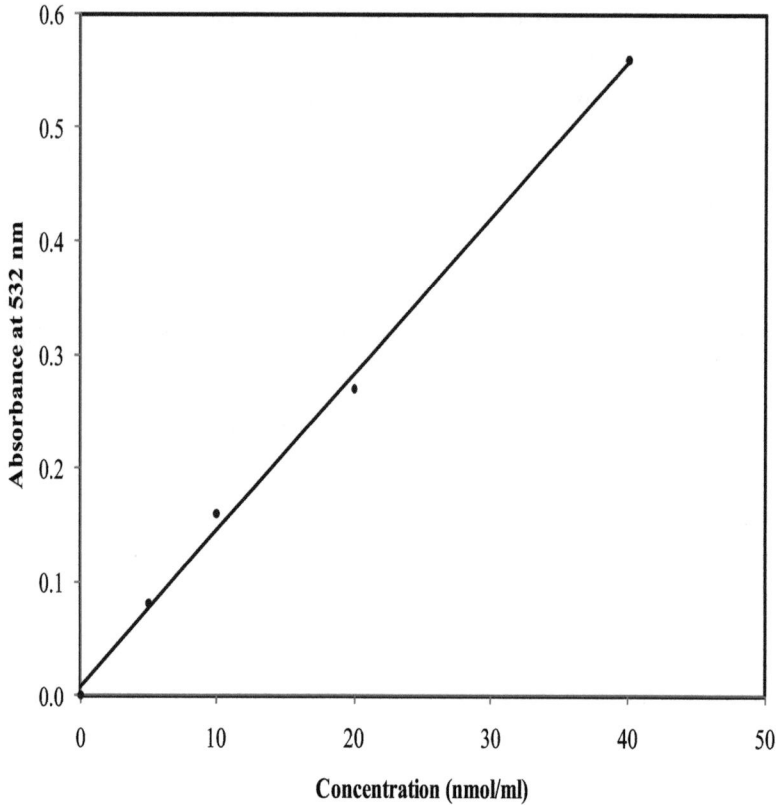

Figure (18): Standard curve of MDA

2-Determination of hepatic reduced glutathione (GSH) [252]

Principle

The GSH was measured according to Murphy's method. This method is based on the reductive cleavage of Ellman's reagent (5,5'-dithiobis-2-nitrobenzoic acid) (DTNB), by SH group of glutathione to yield a yellow color with a maximum absorbance at 412 nm.

$$2GSH + DTNB \rightarrow GSSG + 2\ TNB\ \text{(yellow colored chromophore)}$$

Reagents

1. Trichloroacetic acid (TCA) and disodium salt of ethylene diamine tetraacetic acid (EDTA): disodium salt of EDTA (372 mg) and TCA (50 gm) were dissolved in one liter of distilled water.

2. Solution A: 0.2 M prepared by dissolving 27.8 gm monobasic sodium phosphate (Merck Co, Germany), in one liter of distilled water.

3. Solution B: 0.2 M prepared by dissolving 53.65 gm dibasic sodium phosphate (Merck Co, Germany), in one liter of distilled water.

4. 0.1 M sodium phosphate buffer, pH 8: prepared by adding 26.5 ml of solution A to 473.5 ml of solution B and the volume was adjusted to one liter with distilled water.

5. 0.1 M sodium phosphate buffer, pH 7: prepared by adding 195 ml of solution A to 305 ml of solution B and the volume was adjusted to one liter with distilled water.

6. 0.01 M DTNB: prepared by dissolving 39.5 mg DTNB in 200 ml of 0.1 M sodium phosphate buffer, pH 7.

Procedure

1. The sample was prepared by the addition of an aliquot of 200 μl of the clear supernatant of the 20% liver homogenate in TCA to 4.7 ml of 0.1 M sodium phosphate buffer pH 8, followed by 100 μl of 0.01 M DTNB and vortexed immediately for few seconds.

2. The absorbance of the resultant yellow color was measured spectrophotometerically at 412 nm using Jenway 6305 spectrophotometer within 25 minutes of addition of DTNB against a blank containing 200 µl distilled water instead of the sample.

Calculation

The concentration of reduced glutathione in the liver samples was determined from a standard curve made by preparing serial dilutions of standard reduced glutathione in phosphate buffer pH 8 and treating them as samples, Figure (19).

Results were subsequently expressed as µg reduced glutathione/mg protein by dividing the concentration of glutathione in the sample by the protein concentration in the same sample.

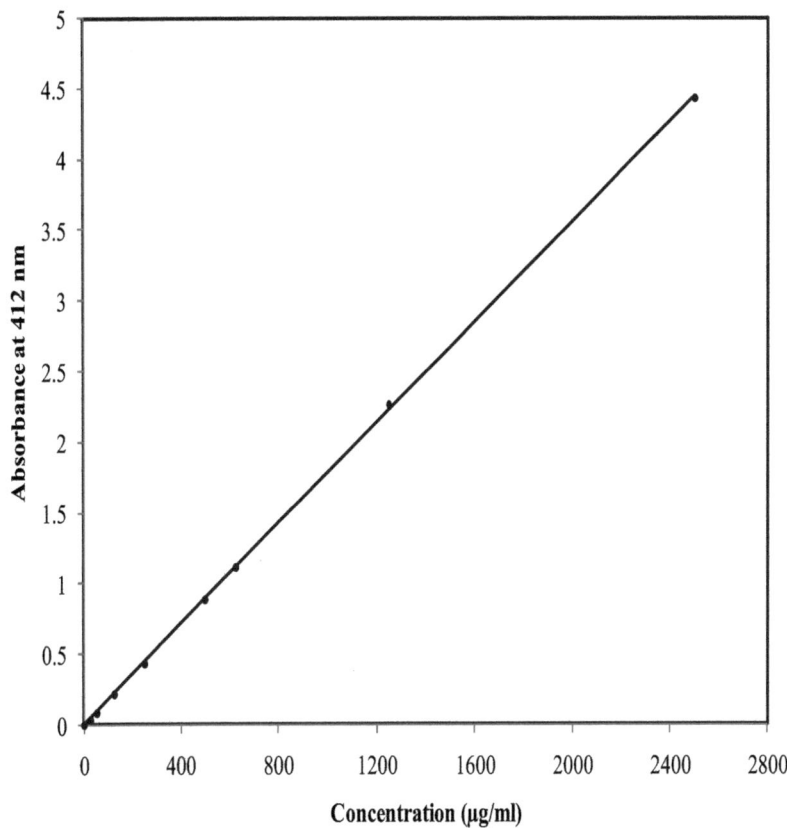

Figure (19): Standard curve of reduced glutathione

3-Determination of total protein [253]

Reaction Principle

Lowry's method was used for the protein determination. The color produced is thought to be due to a complex between the alkaline copper-phenol reagent and tyrosine and tryptophan residues of the protein in the sample. The protein concentration of each sample was estimated by referring to the standard curve constructed using bovine serum albumin fraction V (Sigma Chemical Co, Poole, England).

Reagents

- Sodium hydroxide 0.1 M
- Sodium carbonate (anhydrous) 2% in 0.1 M NaOH
- K^+/Na^+ tartarate 2%
- Copper sulphate 1%
- Lowry C reagent: prepared immediately before use by mixing volumes of sodium carbonate, K^+/Na^+ tartarate and copper sulphate reagent in a ratio 100:1:1
- Folin-Ciocalteau reagent (Sigma Chemical Co, Poole, England). The working reagent was prepared by diluting the stock reagent 1:1 (v/v) with distilled water immediately before use.

Method

The sample was diluted in distilled water (1:10). Aliquots of 10 µl of diluted samples were mixed with 2.5 ml of Lowry C reagent. After incubation 10 minutes at room temperature, 0.25 ml of working Folin-Ciocalteau reagent was added. The tubes were then mixed and incubated in a dark place for one hour at room temperature, after which the absorbance was read at 695 nm using Jenway 6305 spectrophotometer. A blank containing distilled water instead of the sample was treated similarly.

Calculation

The total protein amount was calculated in mg/gm tissue with reference to the protein standard curve, which was constructed by preparing serial concentrations of bovine serum albumin fraction V, Figure (20).

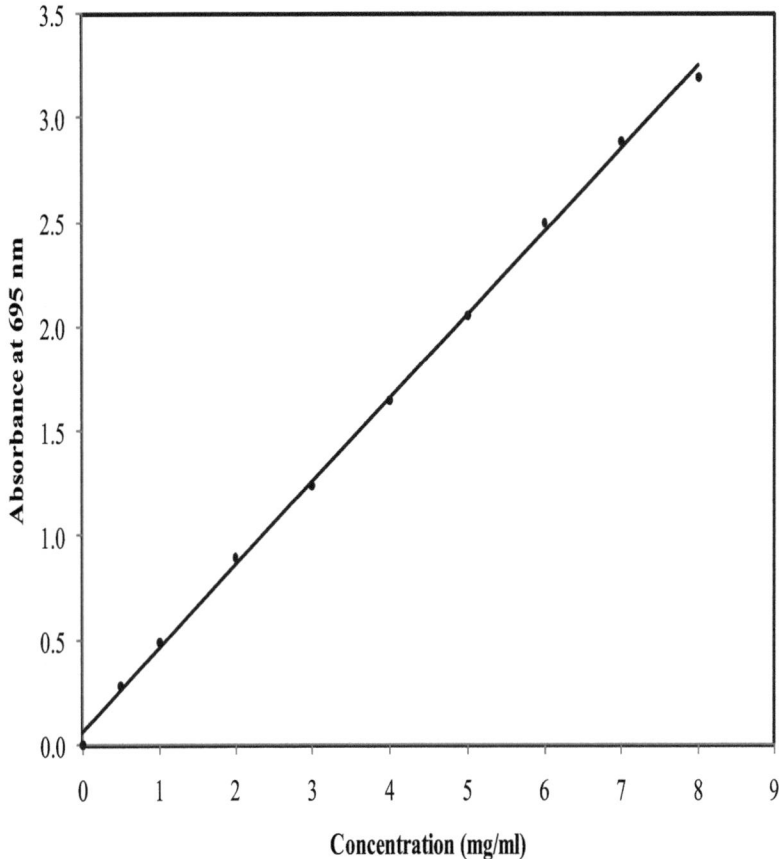

Figure (20): Standard curve of protein

III- Conventional pathological assesment of excised pancreas by Haematoxylin and Eosin (H&E) staining

Excised pancreas were cut into 1-2 cm sections and subjected to the following treatment:

1- Fixation Phase: Formalin (10%) was used as a fixative for 12-24 hours. Fixative prevents autolysis of cells by lysosomal enzymes and protects cells from damage during dehydration and mounting. Fixative also stabilizes the protein skeleton of the cells, giving the cells some structural support to resist deformation and crushing.

2- Dehydration step: it was done by ascending grades of alcohol

3- Embedding step: dehydrated tissues were embedded in a paraffin blocks.

4- Haematoxylin and Eosin (H&E) staining Phase:

Thin sections (3-4 µm) were stained by conventional haematoxylin and eosin (H&E) stain.

   a. Haematoxylin staining for 4 min: Haematoxylin (Genzyme, England) is a salt that dissociates in water into positive and negative ions. Its positive ion (basic-alkaline) readily combines with negatively charged regions of cellular macromolecules, especially phosphate groups of nucleic acids, coloring them blue to purple or black. Any substance, cell or tissue, that tends to be stained in this way by hematoxylin is said to be basophilic. Because of their high nucleic acid (DNA and RNA) content, the nuclei of cells are usually basophilic. However, the cytoplasm of cells is generally not basophilic unless it contains unusually high amounts of RNA (or another macromolecule with appropriate negative charge regions) as, for example, when it is very active in protein synthesis.

   b. Washing with tap water

   c. Eosin staining for 2 min: Eosin water soluble (Chematec, U.K) is also a salt that dissociates in water into ions. Its negative ion, which is acidic in nature, readily combines with positively charged regions of cellular macromolecules, especially positively charged regions of cytoplasmic proteins, coloring them a variety of colors, ranging from pink to red or orange. Any substance, cell or tissue, that tends to be stained in this way by eosin is said to be acidophilic or eosinophilic.

5- Dehydration Phase: Samples were passed in ascending series 70%, 80%, 95%, absolute ethanol for 1 min.

6- Clearing and Dealcoholization Phase: Clearing was performed in equal parts of absolute ethanol and xylene, mixture then followed by two changes of xylene.

7- Mounting Phase: One drop of DPX (Chematec, U.K) was used for mounting. The slides were examined by microscope ZEISS (Axioskop2, Germany), stained sections were examined in all slides and then photographed by camera.

5- Statistical analysis of the data [254, 255]

All values are reported as means ± S.E.M. Statistical comparisons for differences between groups were performed by analysis of variance (ANOVA).Data handling were processed using the microcomputer program statistical package for social science (SPSS) version 18.0 (SPSS, Chicago, IL, USA) [256]. Statistically significant differences were assumed at p value less than 0.05.

1- Arithmetic mean ($\bar{X}$)

This represents the value around which the sum of the deviations of the individual variations have taken plus and minus cancel out, i.e. a measure of central tendency

$$\bar{X} = \frac{\sum(X)}{n}$$

Where:
- $\bar{X}$ = Arithmetic mean
- $\sum(X)$ = sum of values recorded
- n = number of observations

2- The standard deviation (S.D.)

This is used as a measure of dispersion. It was calculated as follows

$$\pm S.D = \sqrt{\frac{\left(\sum X^2\right) - \frac{\left(\sum X\right)^2}{n}}{n-1}}$$

Where:
- $\sum(X^2)$ = Sum of squared values
- $\sum(X)^2$ = Square of the sum of values

3- Standard error of mean (S.E.M.)

This is used as a measure of precision and statistical reliability of the mean, i.e. it is the correction of the standard deviation in relation to the number of observations. It was calculated as follows:

$$\pm S.E.M. = \frac{\pm S.D.}{\sqrt{n}}$$

4- Comparison between more than two groups means (ANOVA) test

F-test (analysis of variance)

This test of significance is used for comparison between more than two groups of variance according to the following equation:

$$F = \frac{\text{Between Group Means Squares (B.M.S)}}{\text{Within Group Mean Squares (W.M.S)}}$$

Where:

$$B.M.S. = \frac{\text{Between Group Sum Squares (B.S.S)}}{(\text{Groups} - 1)}$$

$$B.S.S. = \frac{(\sum X)^2}{K} - \frac{(\sum X)^2}{n}$$

Where :
- K = Number of each group.
- n = Number of samples in all group.

$$W.M.S = \frac{\text{Within Group Sum Squares (W.S.S)}}{n - \text{number of Groups}}$$

$$W.S.S = \sum X^2 - \sum \frac{(\sum X)}{K}$$

5- Least significant difference (L.S.D.)

L.S.D. is used only when F-value was significant to detect the presence of significance between each group.

$$L.S.D = t_{0.05} \sqrt{S_p^2 \left(\frac{1}{n_1} + \frac{1}{n_2} \right)}$$

Where:
- $t_{0.05}$ = The critical value from t-table (2.101).
- n_1 = Number of the first group.
- n_2 = Number of the second group.
- S_p^2 = Pooled variance.

RESULTS

In the present study, the effects of streptozotocin-induced type 2 diabetes in adult male albino rats, on different serum biochemical parameters and hepatic oxidative stress markers are discussed. A summary of the effects obtained after treating diabetic rats with metformin and L-cysteine alone or in combination for 2 weeks on these parameters are also presented.

All results are expressed as mean ± S.E.M.

I- Effect of streptozotocin-induced type 2 diabetes mellitus on the studied parameters in male albino rats

1- Biochemical metabolic parameters

1.1. Fasting serum glucose (FSG)

FSG level was significantly increased in STZ-induced type 2 diabetic rats as compared to normal rats. The mean value of the normal control group was (89.90±2.58 mg/dl) while that of the STZ-rats was (194.40±2.17 mg/dl) at $p< 0.001$. (Table 1) and (Figure 21)

1.2. Fasting serum insulin (FSI)

Type 2 diabetic rats had shown significantly higher values of FSI than the normal control rats at $p< 0.001$. The FSI mean was (4.01±0.09 ng/ml) for the untreated diabetic rats as compared to (1.37±0.04 ng/ml) for the normal rats. (Table 1) and (Figure 22)

1.3. Homeostasis model assessment of insulin resistance (HOMA-IR)

The calculated HOMA-IR mean was (48.13±1.20) in the untreated diabetic group, which showed a statistically significant increase when compared to (7.61±0.29) in the normal control group at $p< 0.001$. (Table 1) and (Figure 23)

2- Lipid profile

The deleterious effects of experimentally-induced type 2 diabetes on lipid profile are shown in table (2) and figure (24A-24G).

2.1. Serum triglycerides (TGs)

Mean value of serum triglycerides was significantly increased in the diabetic untreated rats in comparison to the normal non-diabetic controls at $p< 0.001$. The mean value of triglycerides for normal controls was (39.10±2.03 mg/dl), while that of the untreated diabetic rats was (162.80±1.81 mg/dl). (Table 2) and (Figure 24a)

2.2. Serum total cholesterol (TC)

The present study revealed that there was a significant increase in total cholesterol level in STZ-diabetic rats with a mean value (126.10±1.70 mg/dl) as compared to the normal group in which the mean value was (79.70±1.41 mg/dl) at $p< 0.001$. (Table 2) and (Figure 24b)

2.3. Serum high-density lipoprotein cholesterol (HDL-C)

There was a significant decrease in the mean value of HDL-C of the untreated diabetic group (28.0±0.77 mg/dl) when compared to the mean of the normal controls (58.0±1.15 mg/dl) at $p< 0.001$. (Table 2) and (Figure 24c)

2.4. Serum low-density lipoproteins cholesterol (LDL-C)

Serum LDL-C was significantly increased in STZ-diabetic untreated rats with a mean value of (65.54±0.87 mg/dl) as compared to the mean value (13.88 ±0.82 mg/dl) for the normal controls at $p< 0.001$. (Table 2) and (Figure 24d)

2.5. Serum free fatty acids (FFAs)

The mean value of FFAs in the untreated diabetic rats was significantly higher than that in the normal group at $p< 0.001$. The FFAs mean value was (1.32±0.03 mmol/L) for the untreated diabetic rats as compared to (0.27±0.03 mmol/L) for the normal non-diabetic rats. (Table 2) and (Figure 24e)

2.6. Non-HDL-cholesterol

Experimental STZ-induced diabetes resulted in significantly elevated values of the calculated non-HDL-C at $p< 0.001$. Non-HDL-C mean value increased significantly from (21.70 ± 1.03 mg/dl) in normal rats to (98.10 ± 0.92 mg/dl) in diabetic rats. (Table 2) and (Figure 24f)

2.7. Triglycerides to HDL-cholesterol ratio (TGs/HDL)

The untreated STZ-diabetic rats had shown higher mean value of TGs/HDL ratio (5.85 ± 0.06), as compared to the mean value (0.68 ± 0.15) in the normal group at $p< 0.001$. (Table 2) and (Figure 24g)

3- Hepatic oxidative stress parameters

3.1. Hepatic malondialdehyde (MDA)

As shown in Table (3) and Figure (25), STZ-induced type 2 diabetes resulted in a pro-oxidant state manifested by a significant increase in lipid peroxidation products estimated as hepatic MDA (24.76 ± 0.57 nmol/gm wet tissue) as compared to normal non-diabetic control rats with a mean value of (9.12 ± 0.37 nmol/gm wet tissue) at $p< 0.001$.

3.2. Hepatic reduced glutathione (GSH)

The hepatic GSH content in the untreated diabetic rats, expressed in ratio to total protein content, was significantly lower than normal control rats (135.31 ± 1.64 μg/mg protein versus 250.10 ± 2.31 μg/mg protein) at $p< 0.001$. (Table 3) and (Figure 26)

4- Serum inflammatory parameters

4.1. Monocyte chemoattractant protein-1 (MCP-1)

Experimentally-induced type 2 diabetic rats showed a significantly increased level of serum monocyte chemoattractant protein-1 when compared to the normal control rats at $p< 0.001$. The mean value of MCP-1 for the normal non-diabetic group was (157.84 ± 2.60 pg/ml) while that of the untreated diabetic group was (670.42 ± 9.01 pg/ml). (Table 4) and (Figure 27)

4.2. Serum C-reactive protein (CRP)

Mean value of C-reactive protein was significantly increased in the untreated diabetic rats as compared to the normal non-diabetic controls with mean values (3.25±0.08 mg/L) and (0.40±0.03 mg/L) respectively at p< 0.001. (Table 4) and (Figure 28)

4.3. Serum nitric oxide (NO)

Untreated diabetic rats had shown significantly higher values of serum nitric oxide than the normal control rats at p< 0.001. The NO mean was (65.95±2.07 nmol/ml) for the untreated diabetic rats as compared to (18.77±0.62 nmol/ml) for the normal non-diabetic control rats. (Table 4) and (Figure 29)

Table (1): Effect of STZ-induced type 2 diabetes on fasting serum glucose, fasting serum insulin and HOMA-IR in male albino rats

	Fasting serum glucose (mg/dl)		Fasting serum insulin (ng/ml)		HOMA-IR	
	Normal control group	Untreated diabetic group	Normal control group	Untreated diabetic group	Normal control group	Untreated diabetic group
N	10	10	10	10	10	10
X	89.90 ^{a}	194.40 ^{b}	1.37 ^{a}	4.01 ^{b}	7.61 ^{a}	48.13 ^{b}
S.D.	8.16	6.87	0.13	0.30	0.93	3.81
S.E.	2.58	2.17	0.04	0.09	0.29	1.20
t	30.991*		25.651*		32.702*	
p value	< 0.001					

X: Arithmetic mean   N: Number of animals
t: Student t-test
Different superscripts within each raw indicate statistically significant differences between groups at p < 0.001
* : Statistically significant at p ≤ 0.001

Effect of STZ-induced type 2 diabetes on fasting serum glucose, fasting serum insulin and HOMA-IR in male albino rats

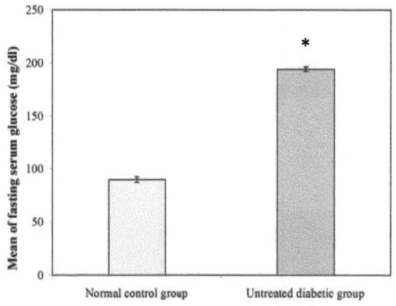

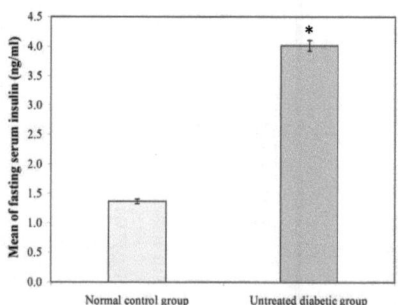

Figure (21): Effect of STZ-induced type 2 diabetes on fasting serum glucose in male albino rats

Figure (22): Effect of STZ-induced type 2 diabetes on fasting serum insulin in male albino rats

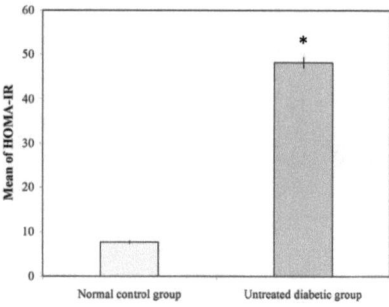

Figure (23): Effect of STZ-induced type 2 diabetes on HOMA-IR in male albino rats

* : Significant in comparison to normal rats

Table (2): Effect of STZ-induced type 2 diabetes on lipid profile in male albino rats

	Triglycerides (mg/dl)		Total cholesterol (mg/dl)		HDL-C (mg/dl)		LDL-C (mg/dl)		Free Fatty Acids (mmol/L)		Non-HDL-C (mg/dl)		TGs/HDL ratio	
	Normal control group	Untreated diabetic group	Normal control group	Untreated diabetic group	Normal control group	Untreated diabetic group	Normal control group	Untreated diabetic group	Normal control group	Untreated diabetic group	Normal control group	Untreated diabetic group	Normal control group	Untreated diabetic group
N	10	10	10	10	10	10	10	10	10	10	10	10	10	10
X	39.10 [a]	162.80 [b]	79.70 [a]	126.10 [b]	58.0 [a]	28.0 [b]	13.88 [a]	65.54 [b]	0.27 [a]	1.32 [b]	21.70 [a]	98.10 [b]	0.68 [a]	5.85 [b]
S.D.	6.42	5.73	4.47	5.36	3.62	2.45	2.59	2.75	0.08	0.09	3.06	3.25	0.13	0.48
S.E.	2.03	1.81	1.41	1.70	1.15	0.77	0.82	0.87	0.03	0.03	1.03	0.92	0.15	0.06
t	45.456*		21.009*		21.701*		43.207*		26.739*		28.051*		17.328*	
p value	<0.001													

X: Arithmetic mean N: Number of animals
t: Student t-test
Different superscripts within each raw indicate statistically significant differences between groups at p < 0.001
* : Statistically significant at $p \leq 0.001$

Effect of STZ-induced type 2 diabetes on lipid profile in male albino rats

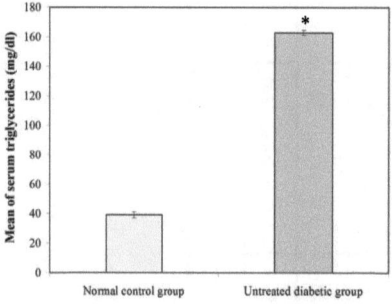

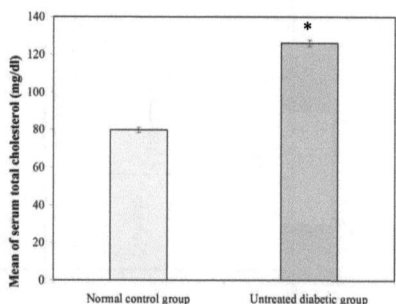

Figure (24a): Effect of STZ-induced type 2 diabetes on serum triglycerides in male albino rats

Figure (24b): Effect of STZ-induced type 2 diabetes on serum total cholesterol in male albino rats

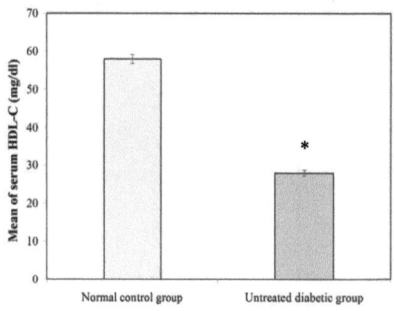

Figure (24c): Effect of STZ-induced type 2 diabetes on serum HDL-C in male albino rats

Figure (24d): Effect of STZ-induced type 2 diabetes on serum LDL-C in male albino rats

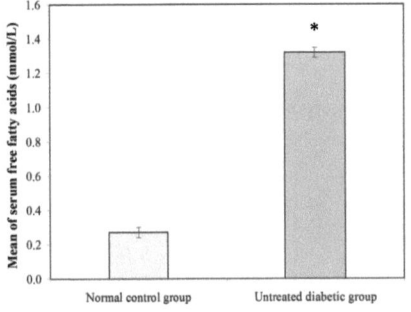 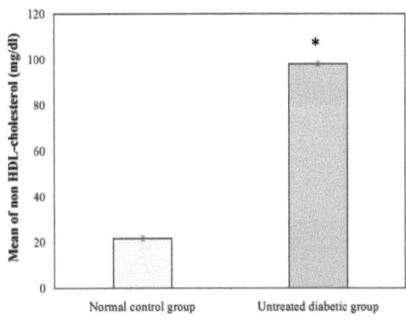

Figure (24e): Effect of STZ-induced type 2 diabetes on serum free fatty acids in male albino rats

Figure (24f): Effect of STZ-induced type 2 diabetes on non-HDL-C in male albino rats

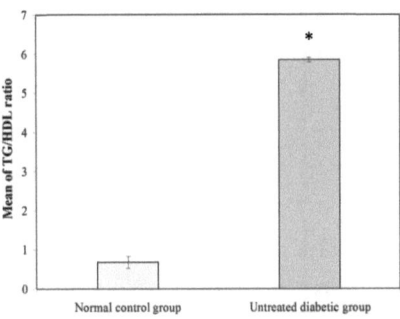

Figure (24g): Effect of STZ-induced type 2 diabetes on TGs/HDL ratio in male albino rats

* : Significant in comparison to normal rats

Table (3): Effect of STZ-induced type 2 diabetes on oxidative stress parameters in male albino rats

	Hepatic malondialdehyde (nmol/gm wet tissue)		Hepatic reduced glutathione (μg/mg protein)	
	Normal control group	Untreated diabetic group	Normal control group	Untreated diabetic group
N	10	10	10	10
X	9.12 [a]	24.76 [b]	250.10 [a]	135.31 [b]
S.D.	1.18	1.80	7.30	5.20
S.E.	0.37	0.57	2.31	1.64
t	23.043*		40.510*	
p value	<0.001			

X: Arithmetic mean N: Number of animals
t: Student t-test
Different superscripts within each raw indicate statistically significant differences between groups at p < 0.001
* : Statistically significant at p ≤ 0.001

Effect of STZ-induced type 2 diabetes on oxidative stress parameters in male albino rats

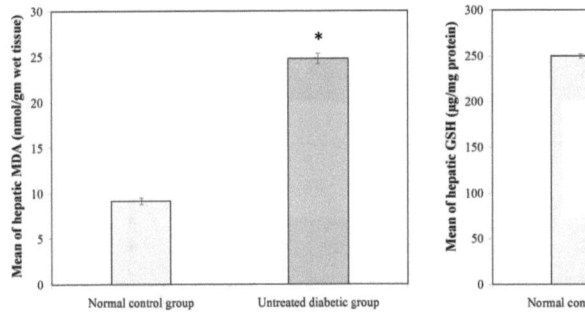
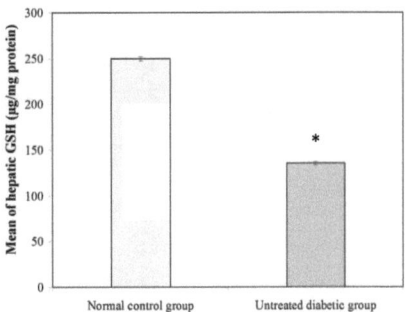

Figure (25): Effect of STZ-induced type 2 diabetes on hepatic malondialdehyde in male albino rats

Figure (26): Effect of STZ-induced type 2 diabetes on hepatic reduced glutathione in male albino rats

* : Significant in comparison to normal rats

Table (4): Effect of STZ-induced type 2 diabetes on inflammatory parameters in male albino rats

	Monocyte chemoattractant protein-1 (pg/ml)		C-reactive protein (mg/L)		Nitric oxide (nmol/L)	
	Normal control group	Untreated diabetic group	Normal control group	Untreated diabetic group	Normal control group	Untreated diabetic group
N	10	10	10	10	10	10
X	157.84 [a]	670.42 [b]	0.40 [a]	3.25 [b]	18.77 [a]	65.95 [b]
S.D.	8.22	28.49	0.09	0.27	1.96	6.56
S.E.	2.60	9.01	0.03	0.08	0.62	2.07
F	54.655*		31.751*		21.803*	
p value	<0.001					

X: Arithmetic mean　　　　N: Number of animals

t: Student t-test

Different superscripts within each raw indicate statistically significant differences between groups at $p < 0.001$

* : Statistically significant at $p \leq 0.001$

Effect of STZ-induced type 2 diabetes on inflammatory parameters in male albino rats

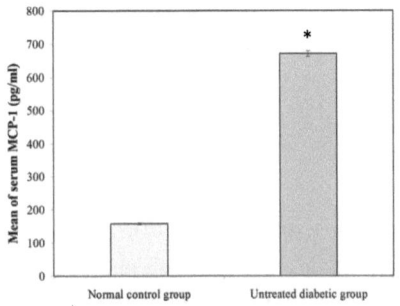
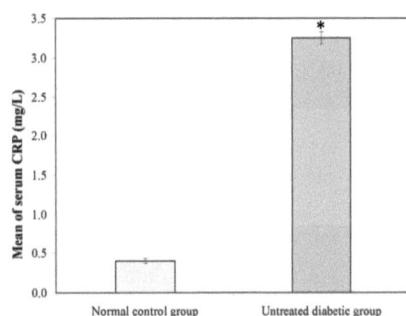

Figure (27): Effect of STZ-induced type 2 diabetes on serum monocyte chemoattractant protein-1 in male albino rats

Figure (28): Effect of STZ-induced type 2 diabetes on serum C-reactive protein in male albino rats

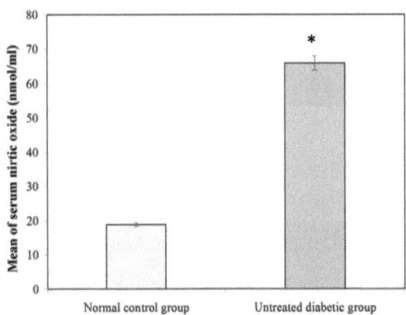

Figure (29): Effect of STZ-induced type 2 diabetes on serum nitric oxide in male albino rats

* : Significant in comparison to normal rats

II- Effect of oral administration of metformin, L-cysteine and their combination for 2 weeks on the studied parameters in STZ-induced male albino rats

1- Biochemical metabolic parameters

1.1. Fasting serum glucose (FSG)

- **Metformin treated group**

Treatment of STZ-induced type 2 diabetic rats with metformin, in a dose of 300 mg/kg/day for 2 weeks orally, was associated with significant decrease in FSG level at $p < 0.001$. The mean values of the FSG were decreased from (194.40 ± 2.17 mg/dl) in the untreated diabetic group to (143.00 ± 1.57 mg/dl) after metformin treatment, (LSD ≥ 7.542). (Table 5) and (Figure 30)

- **L-cysteine treated group**

When L-cysteine was administrated orally in a dose of 300 mg/kg/day for 2 weeks to the STZ-diabetic rats, it resulted in a significant decrease in the mean value of FSG from (194.40 ± 2.17 mg/dl) to (167.20 ± 2.36 mg/dl) at $p < 0.001$, (LSD ≥ 7.542). (Table 5) and (Figure 30)

- **Combination treated group**

Our study revealed that the combination treatment of STZ-induced type 2 diabetes in male albino rats by oral metformin (300 mg/kg/day) and oral L-cysteine (300 mg/kg/day) for 2 weeks caused a significant reduction in the mean value of FSG from (194.40 ± 2.17 mg/dl) to (127.20 ± 1.42 mg/dl) at $p < 0.001$, (LSD ≥ 7.542). (Table 5) and (Figure 30)

Thus both metformin and L-cysteine, alone or in combination, significantly decreased FSG level as compared to untreated diabetic rats at $p < 0.001$. However, the glucose lowering effect of metformin was more evident than that of L-cysteine, as the average values of FSG in the two groups were 26.4% and 14% below the untreated diabetic level, respectively. When both drugs were given in combination, greater decreases in the FSG to about 34.6% below the STZ-diabetic values were observed.

Table (5): Effect of treatment with the studied drugs for 2 weeks on fasting serum glucose in male albino rats (mg/dl)

	Normal control group	Untreated diabetic group	Metformin treated group	L-Cysteine treated group	Combination treated group
N	10	10	10	10	10
X	89.90 [a]	194.40 [b]	143.00 [c]	167.20 [d]	127.20 [e]
S.D.	8.16	6.87	4.97	7.47	4.49
S.E.	2.58	2.17	1.57	2.36	1.42
F			366.806*		
p value			<0.001		
LSD			7.542		

X: Arithmetic mean N: Number of animals
F: F test (ANOVA)
Different superscripts within each raw indicate statistically significant differences between groups at $p < 0.001$
* : Statistically significant at $p \leq 0.001$

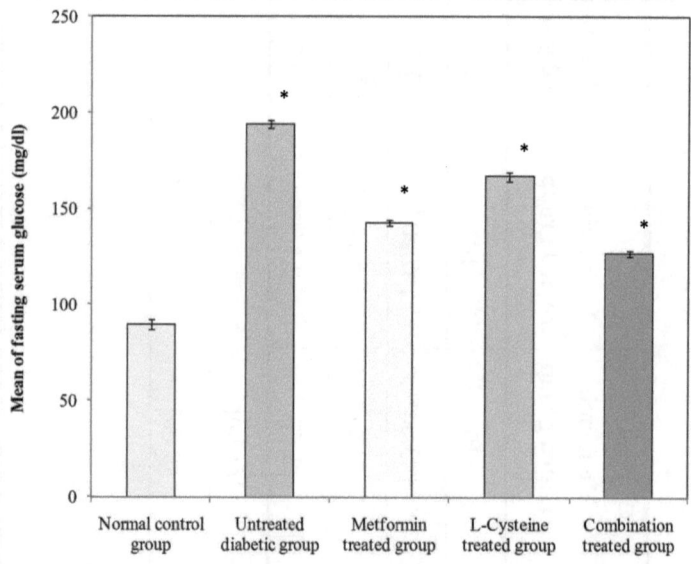

Figure (30): Effect of treatment with the studied drugs for 2 weeks on fasting serum glucose in male albino rats

* : Significant in comparison to normal rats

1.2. Fasting serum insulin (FSI)

• Metformin treated group

Metformin treatment to the STZ-diabetic rats in a dose of 300 mg/kg/day for 2 weeks orally caused a significant decrease in the FSI, reaching a value of (2.64±0.05 ng/ml) as compared to the untreated diabetic group in which the mean value of FSI was (4.01±0.09 ng/ml) at $p< 0.001$, (LSD ≥ 0.205). (Table 6) and (Figure 31)

•L-cysteine treated group

Treating STZ-diabetic rats with oral L-cysteine in a dose of 300 mg/kg/day for 2 weeks significantly reduced the FSI when compared to the untreated group at $p< 0.001$. The mean value of FSI was (3.24±0.04 ng/ml) in the L-cysteine treated group while that of the diabetic group was (4.01±0.09 ng/ml), (LSD ≥ 0.205). (Table 6) and (Figure 31)

• Combination treated group

Concurrent administration of both metformin (300 mg/kg/day) and L-cysteine (300 mg/kg/day) for 2 weeks orally to the STZ-induced diabetic rats reduced that FSI significantly as compared to the untreated diabetic rats with mean values of (2.19±0.03 ng/ml) and (4.01±0.09 ng/ml) respectively, $p< 0.001$, (LSD ≥ 0.205). (Table 6) and (Figure 31)

The effects of both drugs given alone and in combination on FSI were qualitatively similar to their effect on FSG. Treatment with either metformin or L-cysteine alone for 2 weeks resulted in significant decreases in FSI to about 34.2% and 19.2% below the STZ-diabetic values respectively, $p< 0.001$. The reduction of FSI was more evident in the combination group than either drug alone, reaching values 45.4% below the untreated diabetic rats.

Table (6): Effect of treatment with the studied drugs for 2 weeks on fasting serum insulin in male albino rats (ng/ml)

	Normal control group	Untreated diabetic group	Metformin treated group	L-Cysteine treated group	Combination treated group
N	10	10	10	10	10
X	1.37[a]	4.01[b]	2.64[c]	3.24[d]	2.19[e]
S.D.	0.13	0.30	0.15	0.14	0.10
S.E.	0.04	0.09	0.05	0.04	0.03
F	\multicolumn{5}{c}{317.064*}
p value	\multicolumn{5}{c}{<0.001}
LSD	\multicolumn{5}{c}{0.205}

X: Arithmetic mean N: Number of animals
F: F test (ANOVA)
Different superscripts within each raw indicate statistically significant differences between groups at $p < 0.001$
* : Statistically significant at $p \leq 0.001$

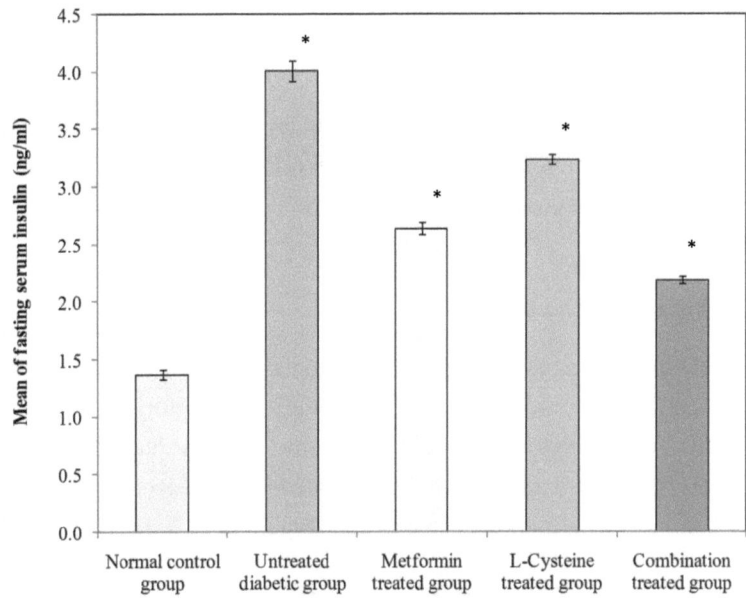

Figure (31): Effect of treatment with the studied drugs for 2 weeks on fasting serum insulin in male albino rats

* : Significant in comparison to normal rats

1.3. Insulin resistance (HOMA-IR)

• Metformin treated group

Treatment with oral metformin in a dose of 300 mg/kg/day for 2 weeks significantly decreased the HOMA-IR mean value to (23.31±0.40) as compared to the mean value of untreated diabetic rats (48.13±1.20) at p< 0.001, (LSD ≥ 2.460). (Table 7) and (Figure 32)

• L-cysteine treated group

Treatment with L-cysteine (300 mg/kg/day) for 2 weeks orally, caused a significant reduction in the HOMA-IR levels (33.41±0.70) in comparison to the STZ-diabetic group (48.13±1.20) at p< 0.001, (LSD ≥ 2.460). (Table 7) and (Figure 32)

• Combination treated group

The study also revealed that the combination oral of metformin (300 mg/kg/day) and oral L-cysteine (300 mg/kg/day) for 2 weeks was associated with a significant decrease in the mean value of HOMA-IR (17.21±0.31) when compared to the untreated diabetic group (48.13±1.20) at p< 0.001, (LSD ≥ 2.460). (Table 7) and (Figure 32)

As presented here, treatments with either metformin or L-cysteine alone or in combination for 2 weeks resulted in significant decreases in HOMA-IR. The mean values of HOMA-IR in the metformin and L-cysteine groups decreased significantly by about 51.6% and 30.6% from the untreated diabetic values respectively, reaching greater significant decreases in the combination treated group, 64.2% below the untreated diabetic rats. All decreases carried a statistical significance at p< 0.001.

Table (7): Effect of treatment with the studied drugs for 2 weeks on HOMA-IR in male albino rats

	Normal control group	Untreated diabetic group	Metformin treated group	L-Cysteine treated group	Combination treated group
N	10	10	10	10	10
X	7.61 [a]	48.13 [b]	23.31 [c]	33.41 [d]	17.21 [e]
S.D.	0.93	3.81	1.28	2.21	0.97
S.E.	0.29	1.20	0.40	0.70	0.31
F			530.376*		
p value			<0.001		
LSD			2.460		

X: Arithmetic mean   N: Number of animals

F: F test (ANOVA)

Different superscripts within each raw indicate statistically significant differences between groups at $p < 0.001$

* : Statistically significant at $p \leq 0.001$

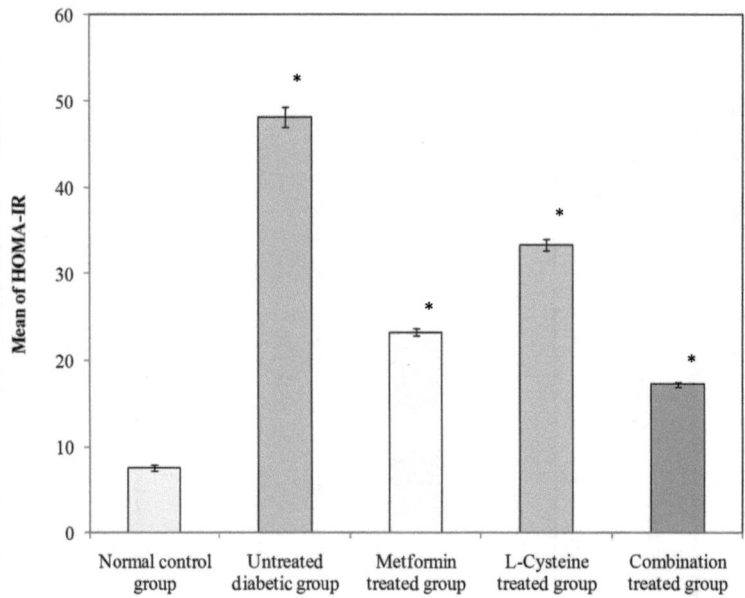

Figure (32): Effect of treatment with the studied drugs for 2 weeks on HOMA-IR in male albino rats

* : Significant in comparison to normal rat

2- Lipid profile

2.1. Serum triglycerides (TGs)

- **Metformin treated group**

In the metformin treated group, given metformin orally in a dose of 300 mg/kg/day for 2 weeks, the mean value of the serum TGs was (122.60±1.065 mg/dl), which was significantly less than that of the untreated diabetic rats (162.80±1.81 mg/dl) at $p < 0.001$, (LSD $\geq$ 5.732). (Table 8) and (Figure 33a)

- **L-cysteine treated group**

Treatment of diabetic rats with L-cysteine in a dose of 300 mg/kg/day for 2 weeks orally resulted in a non-significant decrease in serum TGs as compared to the untreated diabetic rats. The mean values of both groups were (157.50±1.06 mg/dl) and (162.80±1.81 mg/dl) respectively at $p > 0.05$, (LSD < 5.732). (Table 8) and (Figure 33a)

- **Combination treated group**

Treatment of STZ-diabetic rats with both metformin (300 mg/kg/day) and L-cysteine (300 mg/kg/day) for 2 weeks orally was associated with a significant reduction in the mean value of serum TGs (118.50±1.07 mg/dl) when compared to the untreated diabetic rats with mean value of (162.80±1.81 mg/dl) at $p < 0.001$, (LSD $\geq$ 5.732). (Table 8) and (Figure 33a)

Thus, metformin treatment alone caused a statistically significant reduction in serum triglycerides reaching values of 24.7% below STZ-diabetic rats, $p < 0.001$. This decrease in the combination treated group was quantitatively similar to the metformin group, as the mean value of serum triglycerides was 27.2% below diabetic values without significant differences between the two groups. In the L-cysteine group, the level of serum triglycerides was not significantly affected as they decreased by only 3.3% from untreated diabetic values.

Table (8): Effect of treatment with the studied drugs for 2 weeks on serum triglycerides in male albino rats (mg/dl)

	Normal control group	Untreated diabetic group	Metformin treated group	L-Cysteine treated group	Combination treated group
N	10	10	10	10	10
X	39.10 [a]	162.80 [b]	122.60 [c]	157.50 [b]	118.50 [c]
S.D.	6.42	5.73	5.21	3.34	3.37
S.E.	2.03	1.81	1.065	1.06	1.07
F	988.944*				
p value	<0.001				
LSD	5.732				

X: Arithmetic mean　　　　N: Number of animals
F: F test (ANOVA)
Different superscripts within each raw indicate statistically significant differences between groups at $p < 0.001$
* : Statistically significant at $p \leq 0.001$

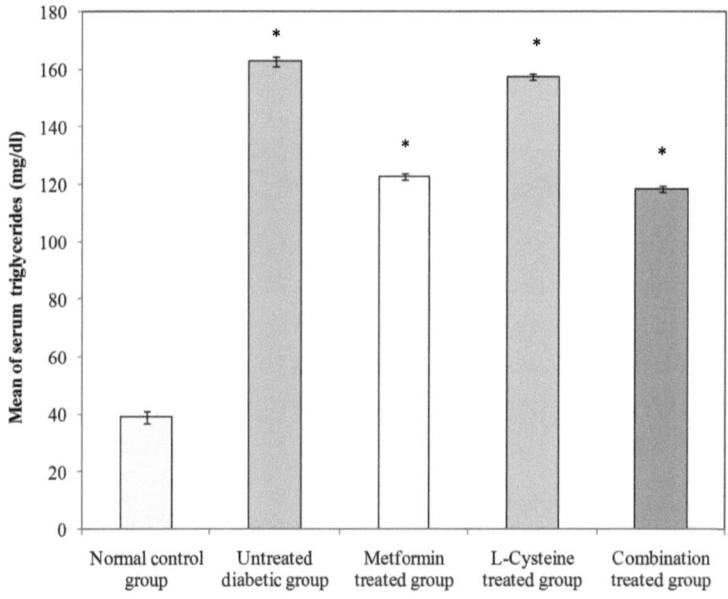

Figure (33a): Effect of treatment with the studied drugs for 2 weeks on serum triglycerides in male albino rats

* : Significant in comparison to normal rats

2.2. Serum total cholesterol (TC)

• Metformin treated group

Treating STZ-diabetic rats with oral metformin in a dose of 300 mg/kg/day for 2 weeks caused a significant decrease in the mean value of total cholesterol to (99.60±1.12 mg/dl) when compared to the untreated diabetic rats (126.10±1.70 mg/dl) at $p< 0.001$, (LSD $\geq$ 4.940). (Table 9) and (Figure 33b)

• L-cysteine treated group

A non-significant decrease in the mean value of total cholesterol resulted by L-cysteine treatment given orally in a dose of 300 mg/kg/day for 2 weeks as compared to the untreated STZ-diabetic rats at $p> 0.05$. The mean value of L-cysteine treated group was (121.20±0.88 mg/dl) while that of the STZ-diabetic group was (126.10±1.70 mg/dl), (LSD < 4.940). (Table 9) and (Figure 33b)

• Combination treated group

Combination treatment of metformin in a dose of 300 mg/kg/day and L-cysteine in a dose of 300 mg/kg/day, given orally for 2 weeks to STZ-diabetic rats, showed a significant decrease in the mean level of total cholesterol from a value of (126.10±1.70 mg/dl) in the untreated diabetic group to reach a value of (96.50±1.02 mg/dl) after treatment at $p< 0.001$, (LSD $\geq$ 4.940). (Table 9) and (Figure 33b)

As resulted in serum triglycerides, metformin treated group and combination treated group showed a quantitatively similar decreases in the serum total cholesterol level, without statistically significant differences between the two groups. The mean values of total cholesterol in both groups were 21% and 23.5% below the untreated diabetic value, respectively. While L-cysteine treated group showed a non-significant decrease in the serum total cholesterol mean value, as it only caused 3.9% decrease from the untreated diabetic value.

Table (9): Effect of treatment with the studied drugs for 2 weeks on serum total cholesterol in male albino rats (mg/dl)

	Normal control group	Untreated diabetic group	Metformin treated group	L-Cysteine treated group	Combination treated group
N	10	10	10	10	10
X	79.70 [a]	126.10 [b]	99.60 [c]	121.20 [b]	96.50 [c]
S.D.	4.47	5.36	3.53	2.78	3.24
S.E.	1.41	1.70	1.12	0.88	1.02
F			227.740*		
p value			<0.001		
LSD			4.940		

X: Arithmetic mean N: Number of animals
F: F test (ANOVA)
Different superscripts within each raw indicate statistically significant differences between groups at $p < 0.001$
*: Statistically significant at $p \leq 0.001$

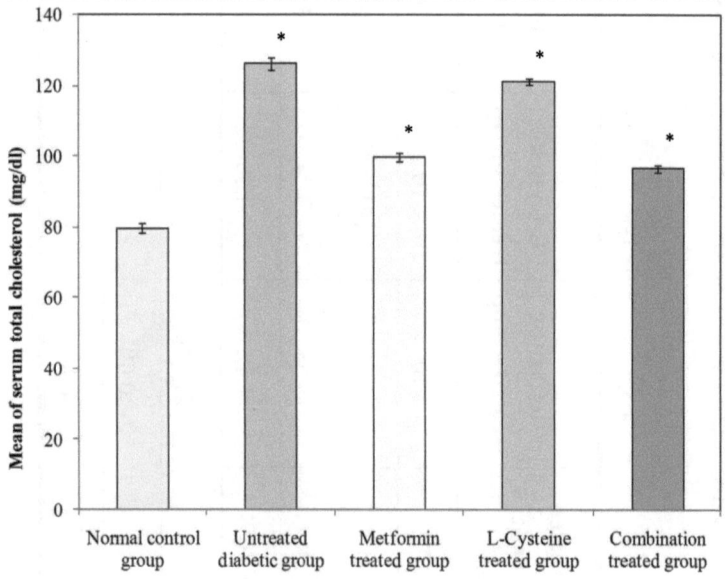

Figure (33b): Effect of treatment with the studied drugs for 2 weeks on serum total cholesterol in male albino rats

* : Significant in comparison to normal rats

2.3. Serum high-density lipoprotein cholesterol (HDL-C)

- **Metformin treated group**

Oral metformin treatment (300 mg/kg/day for 2 weeks) significantly increased the mean level of serum HDL-C (40.20±0.77 mg/dl) as compared to the mean value of the untreated diabetic rats, which was (28.0±0.77 mg/dl) at $p< 0.001$, (LSD ≥ 3.069). (Table 10) and (Figure 33c)

- **L-cysteine treated group**

Oral L-cysteine in a dose 300 mg/kg/day for 2 weeks produced a significant increase in the mean value of serum HDL-C in comparison to the untreated diabetic rats with mean values of (34.10±0.80 mg/dl) and (28.0±0.77 mg/dl), respectively at $p< 0.001$, (LSD ≥ 3.069). (Table 10) and (Figure 33c)

- **Combination treated group**

Treatment of STZ-rats with oral metformin (300 mg/kg/day) in combination with oral L-cysteine (300 mg/kg/day) for 2 weeks caused a significant increase in serum HDL-C mean value (45.90±0.64 mg/dl) when compared to (28.0±0.77 mg/dl) in the diabetic group at $p< 0.001$, (LSD ≥ 3.069). (Table 10) and (Figure 33c)

Thus, the serum HDL-C mean value was greatly increased in the metformin treated group to about 143.6% that of untreated diabetic rats, $p< 0.001$. L-cysteine treatment caused less significant increases in serum HDL-C as compared to the metformin treated group reaching an average of 121.8% of diabetic value, $p< 0.001$. Moreover, the increase in serum HDL-C was even higher in the combination treated group, increasing up to 163.9% of STZ-diabetic value.

Table (10): Effect of treatment with the studied drugs for 2 weeks on serum HDL-C in male albino rats (mg/dl)

	Normal control group	Untreated diabetic group	Metformin treated group	L-Cysteine treated group	Combination treated group
N	10	10	10	10	10
X	58.0 [a]	28.0 [b]	40.20 [c]	34.10 [d]	45.90 [e]
S.D.	3.62	2.45	2.44	2.51	2.02
S.E.	1.15	0.77	0.77	0.80	0.64
F			186.68*		
p value			<0.001		
LSD			3.069		

X: Arithmetic mean N: Number of animal
F: F test (ANOVA)
Different superscripts within each raw indicate statistically significant differences between groups at $p < 0.001$
* : Statistically significant at $p \leq 0.001$

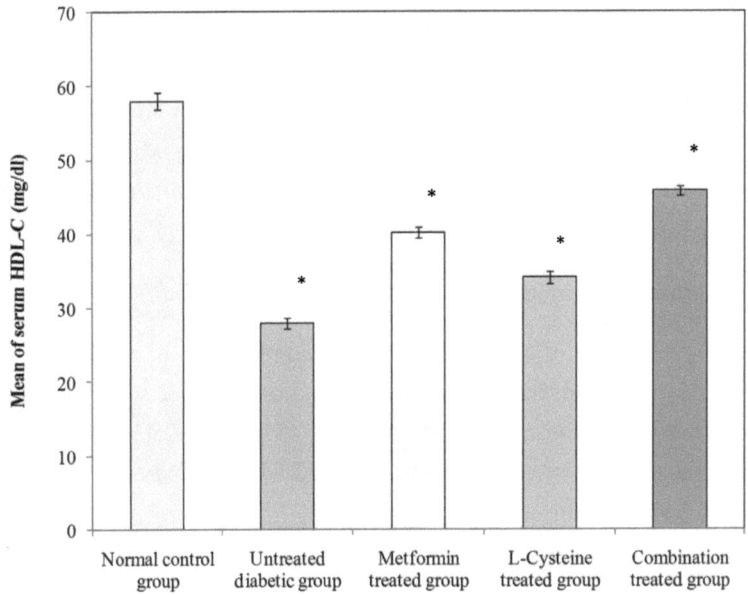

Figure (33c): Effect of treatment with the studied drugs for 2 weeks on serum high-density lipoprotein cholesterol in male albino rats

* : Significant in comparison to normal rats

2.4. Serum low-density lipoprotein cholesterol (LDL-C)

- **Metformin treated group**

A dose of 300 mg/kg/day of oral metformin given to the STZ-diabetic rats for 2 weeks resulted in a significant reduction in the LDL-C mean value to reach (34.88±0.85 mg/dl) in comparison to the untreated diabetic group mean value, which was (65.54±0.87 mg/dl) at $p< 0.001$, (LSD $\geq$ 2.887). (Table 11) and (Figure 33d)

- **L-cysteine treated group**

Treatment with oral L-cysteine (300 mg/kg/day) for 2 weeks was associated with a significant decrease in the mean value of LDL-C (55.60±0.90 mg/dl) as compared to (65.54±0.87 mg/dl) in the untreated diabetic rats at $p< 0.001$, (LSD $\geq$ 2.887). (Table 11) and (Figure 33d)

- **Combination treated group**

The treatment of diabetic rats with a combination of metformin (300 mg/kg/day) and L-cysteine (300 mg/kg/day) orally for 2 weeks decreased significantly the mean level of LDL-C to (26.90±0.43 mg/dl) when compared to the untreated diabetic rats (65.54±0.87 mg/dl) at $p< 0.001$, (LSD $\geq$ 2.887). (Table 11) and (Figure 33d)

Therefore, metformin treatment for 2 weeks caused a significant decrease in serum LDL-C averaging 46.8% below the untreated diabetic values, $p< 0.001$. In the L-cysteine group, less but significant reduction in LDL-C was observed, reaching value of about 15.2% below STZ-diabetic value, $p< 0.001$. The combined effect of both drugs on serum LDL-C was more profound than either drug alone, as its level significantly decreased by about 59% from untreated diabetic rats, $p< 0.001$.

Table (11): Effect of treatment with the studied drugs for 2 weeks on serum LDL-C in male albino rats (mg/dl)

	Normal control group	Untreated diabetic group	Metformin treated group	L-Cysteine treated group	Combination treated group
N	10	10	10	10	10
X	13.88 ^{a}	65.54 ^{b}	34.88 ^{c}	55.60 ^{d}	26.90 ^{e}
S.D.	2.59	2.75	2.68	2.83	1.37
S.E.	0.82	0.87	0.85	0.90	0.43
F			706.044*		
p value			<0.001		
LSD			2.887		

X: Arithmetic mean   N: Number of animals
F: F test (ANOVA)
Different superscripts within each raw indicate statistically significant differences between groups at $p < 0.001$
* : Statistically significant at $p \leq 0.001$

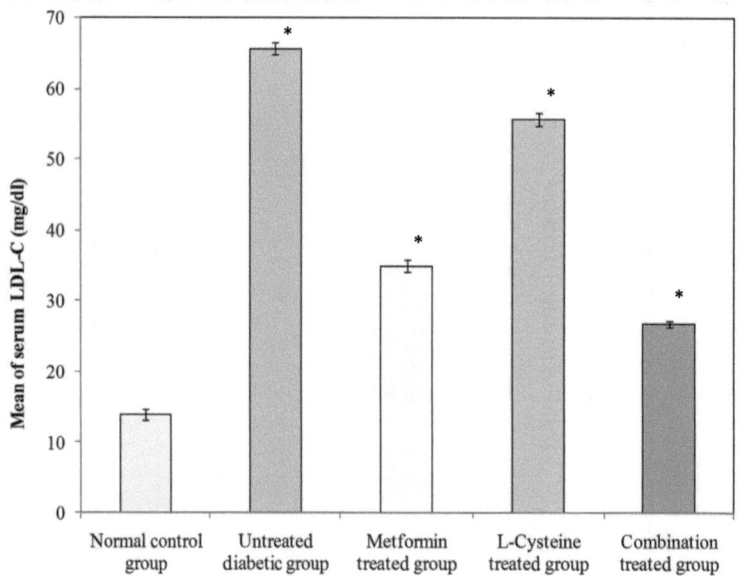

Figure (33d): Effect of treatment with the studied drugs for 2 weeks on serum low-density lipoprotein cholesterol in male albino rats

* : Significant in comparison to normal rats

2.5. Serum Free fatty acids (FFAs)

• Metformin treated group

When metformin administrated orally to the STZ-diabetic rats in a dose 300 mg/kg/day for 2 weeks, it caused a significant decrease in the mean value of FFAs (0.66 ± 0.02 mmol/L) as compared to (1.32 ± 0.03 mmol/L) in the untreated diabetic rats at $p < 0.001$, (LSD ≥ 0.087). (Table 12) and (Figure 33e)

• L-cysteine treated group

The oral administration of L-cysteine in a dose of 300 mg/kg/day for 2 weeks significantly decreased the FFAs mean value to reach (0.89 ± 0.03 mmol/L) in comparison to the mean value in untreated diabetic group, which was (1.32 ± 0.03 mmol/L) at $p < 0.001$, (LSD ≥ 0.087). (Table 12) and (Figure 33e)

• Combination treated group

Concurrent treatment with both metformin (300 mg/kg/ day) and L-cysteine (300 mg/kg/day) for 2 weeks orally was associated with a significant reduction in the mean value of FFAs when compared to the untreated STZ-diabetic rats at $p < 0.001$. The FFAs mean values in both groups were (0.50 ± 0.01 mmol/L) and (1.32 ± 0.03 mmol/L) respectively, (LSD ≥ 0.087). (Table 12) and (Figure 33e)

As shown, treatment with either metformin or L-cysteine alone for 2 weeks caused significant decreases in the mean value of FFAs to reach 50% and 32.6% below the values of the untreated diabetic rats, respectively, $p < 0.001$. Meanwhile, the combination between both drugs resulted in a more evident reduction in FFAs level, reaching about 62.1% below STZ-diabetic value, $p < 0.001$.

Table (12): Effect of treatment with the studied drugs for 2 weeks on serum free fatty acids in male albino rats (mmol/L)

	Normal control group	Untreated diabetic group	Metformin treated group	L-Cysteine treated group	Combination treated group
N	10	10	10	10	10
X	0.27 [a]	1.32 [b]	0.66 [c]	0.89 [d]	0.50 [e]
S.D.	0.08	0.09	0.06	0.09	0.04
S.E.	0.03	0.03	0.02	0.03	0.01
F			282.279*		
p value			<0.001		
LSD			0.087		

X: Arithmetic mean N: Number of animals
F: F test (ANOVA)
Different superscripts within each raw indicate statistically significant differences between groups at $p < 0.001$
* : Statistically significant at $p \leq 0.001$

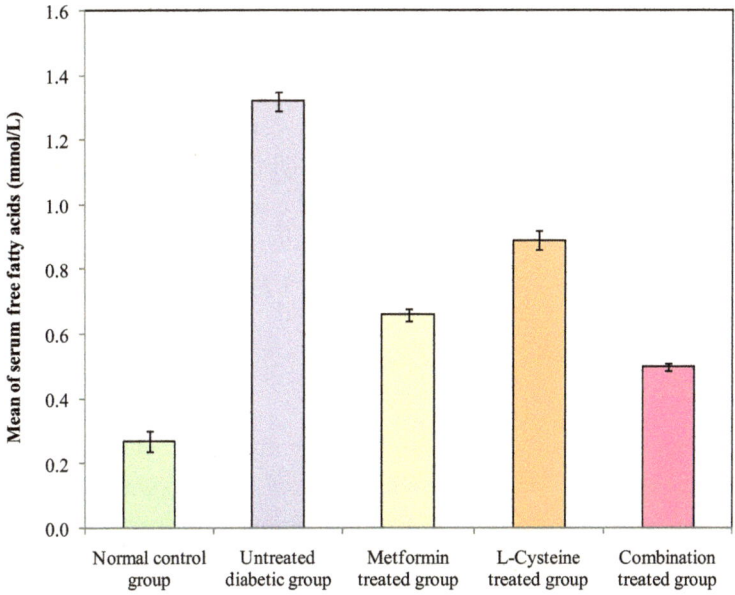

Figure (33e): Effect of treatment with the studied drugs for 2 weeks on serum free fatty acids in male albino rats

* : Significant in comparison to normal rats

2.6. Non-HDL-cholesterol

• Metformin treated group

Metformin treatment, given in a dose of 300 mg/kg/day for 2 weeks orally, resulted in a significant reduction in the non-HDL-C mean values (59.40±0.95 mg/dl) when compared to (98.1±0.92 mg/dl) in the untreated STZ-diabetic rats at p< 0.001, (LSD ≥ 3.243). (Table 13) and (Figure 33f)

• L-cysteine treated group

Treatment of STZ-diabetic rats with L-cysteine in a dose of 300 mg/kg/day for 2 weeks orally caused a significant decrease in the mean value of non-HDL-C when compared to the untreated diabetic rats at p< 0.001. The mean values of the both groups were (87.10±0.48 mg/ dl) and (98.10±0.92 mg/ dl) respectively, (LSD ≥ 3.243). (Table 13) and (Figure 33f)

• Combination treated group

The current study revealed that the combination between metformin and L-cysteine, both given orally in a dose of 300 mg/kg/day for 2 weeks, was associated with a significant reduction in the mean value of the calculated non-HDL-C, reaching a value of (50.60±0.97 mg/dl) as compared to the untreated diabetic mean value, which was (98.10±0.92 mg/dl) at p< 0.001, (LSD ≥ 3.243). (Table 13) and (Figure 33f)

Therefore, metformin treatment alone resulted in a more significant decrease in the mean value of non-HDL-C as compared to the L-cysteine group, p< 0.001. Non-HDL-C mean values in both groups were 39.4% and 11.2% below the untreated diabetic value, respectively. Such decreases were more significant in the combination treated group, reaching average value of 48.4% below the untreated diabetic value.

Table (13): Effect of treatment with the studied drugs for 2 weeks on non-HDL-cholesterol in male albino rats (mg/dl)

	Normal control group	untreated diabetic group	Metformin treated group	L-Cysteine treated group	Combination treated group
N	10	10	10	10	10
X	21.70 [a]	98.10 [b]	59.40 [c]	87.10 [d]	50.60 [e]
S.D.	3.06	3.25	2.91	3.0	1.51
S.E.	1.03	0.92	0.95	0.48	0.97
F	1162.061 *				
p value	<0.001				
LSD	3.243				

X: Arithmetic mean   N: Number of animals

F: F test (ANOVA)

Different superscripts within each raw indicate statistically significant differences between groups at $p < 0.001$

* : Statistically significant at $p \leq 0.001$

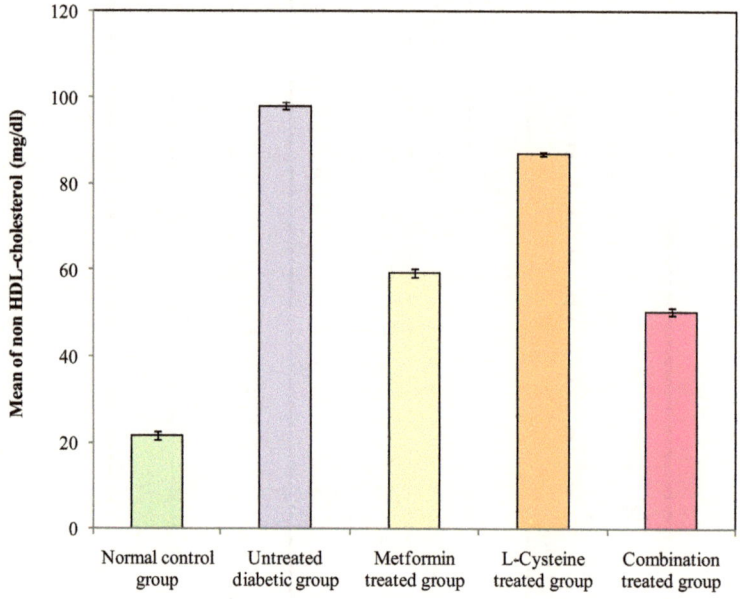

Figure (33f): Effect of treatment with the studied drugs for 2 weeks on non-HDL-cholesterol in male albino rats

* : Significant in comparison to normal rats

2.7. Triglycerides to HDL-cholesterol ratio (TGs/HDL)

• Metformin treated group

There was a significant decrease in TGs/HDL ratio in rats treated with metformin, in a dose of 300 mg/kg/day for 2 weeks orally, to reach a mean value of (3.06±0.13) in comparison with the untreated diabetic rats with a mean value of (5.85±0.06) at $p< 0.001$, (LSD $\geq$ 0.342). (Table 14) and (Figure 33g)

• L-cysteine treated group

It was also observed that treatment of diabetic rats with L-cysteine, in the previously mentioned dose, was associated with a significant decrease in TGs/HDL ratio when compared to the STZ-diabetic rats at $p< 0.001$. The mean values of both groups were (4.65±0.03) and (5.85±0.06) respectively, (LSD $\geq$ 0.342). (Table 14) and (Figure 33g)

• Combination treated group:

The results revealed that the combination treatment between metformin in a dose of 300 mg/kg/day and L-cysteine in a dose of 300 mg/kg/day for 2 weeks orally reduced significantly the mean value of TGs/HDL ratio to (2.58±0.04) as compared to (5.85±0.06) in the untreated diabetic rats at $p< 0.001$, (LSD $\geq$ 0.342). (Table 14) and (Figure 33g)

Thus, it was concluded that metformin treatment caused a more significant reduction in the level of TGs/HDL ratio in comparison to the L-cysteine treated group, reaching values about 47.7% and 20.5% below the untreated diabetic value, respectively at $p< 0.001$. Such decrease in the level of TGs/HDL ratio was more significant in the combination treated group, reaching average value of 55.9% below the STZ-diabetic value.

Table (14): Effect of treatment with the studied drugs for 2 weeks on triglycerides to HDL-cholesterol ratio in male albino rats

	Normal control group	untreated diabetic group	Metformin treated group	L-Cysteine treated group	Combination treated group
N	10	10	10	10	10
X	0.68[a]	5.85[b]	3.06[c]	4.65[d]	2.58[e]
S.D.	0.13	0.48	0.18	0.40	0.08
S.E.	0.15	0.06	0.13	0.03	0.04
F			446.129*		
p value			<0.001		
LSD			0.342		

X: Arithmetic mean N: Number of animals
F: F test (ANOVA)
Different superscripts within each raw indicate statistically significant differences between groups at $p < 0.001$
* : Statistically significant at $p \leq 0.001$

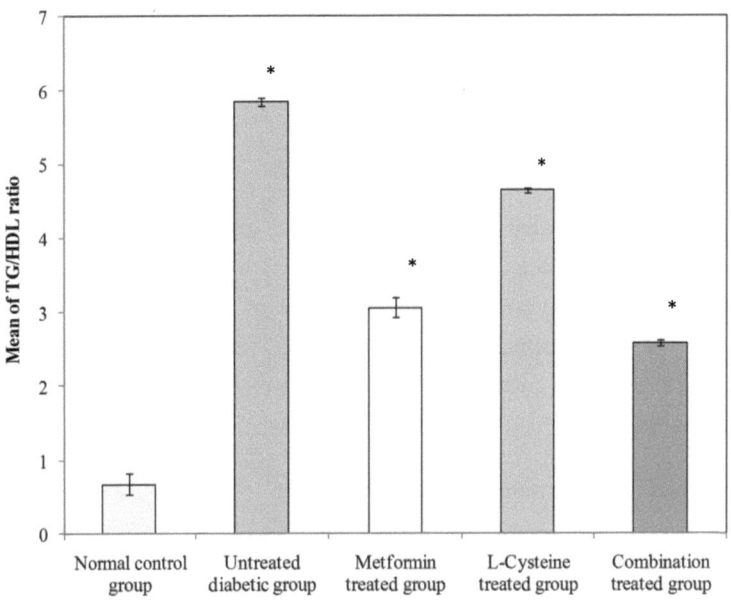

Figure (33g): Effect of treatment with the studied drugs for 2 weeks on triglycerides to HDL-cholesterol ratio in male albino rats

* : Significant in comparison to normal rats

3. Hepatic oxidative stress parameters

3.1. Hepatic malondialdehyde (MDA)

• **Metformin treated group**

The hepatic MDA in STZ-diabetic rats treated with metformin in a dose of 300 mg/kg/day orally for 2 weeks was significantly lower than that of the untreated diabetic rats at $p< 0.001$. The mean values of both groups were (18.69±0.37 nmol/gm wet tissue) and (24.76±0.57 nmol/gm wet tissue) respectively, (LSD ≥ 1.403). (Table 15) and (Figure 34)

• **L-cysteine treated group**

Treating STZ-diabetic rats with oral L-cysteine, in a dose of 300 mg/kg/day for 2 weeks significantly reduced the increased hepatic MDA levels seen in the untreated diabetic rats at $p< 0.001$. The hepatic MDA mean value was decreased from (24.76±0.57 nmol/gm wet tissue) in the untreated diabetic group to (15.44±0.20 nmol/gm wet tissue) after L-cysteine treatment, (LSD ≥ 1.403). (Table 15) and (Figure 34)

• **Combination treated group**

According to the data presented in Table 15 and Figure 34, oral metformin (300 mg/kg/day) and oral L-cysteine (300 mg/kg/day), given together for 2 weeks, significantly decreased the hepatic MDA levels to (12.78±0.33 nmol/gm wet tissue) as compared to the MDA mean value (24.76±0.57 nmol/gm wet tissue) in the untreated diabetic group at $p< 0.001$, (LSD ≥ 1.403).

Thus, it was observed that the concentration of hepatic MDA in the metformin treated group decreased significantly to approximately 76% of untreated diabetic values. The reduction in MDA level was more evident in the L-cysteine group, reaching an average of 62.4% of diabetic values. However, treatment of diabetic rats with metformin and L-cysteine in combination decreased MDA levels more significantly than either drug alone, to reach an average MDA value about 51% that of the untreated diabetic rats. All decreases carried a statistical significance at $p< 0.001$.

Table (15): Effect of treatment with the studied drugs for 2 weeks on hepatic malondialdehyde in male albino rats (nmol/gm wet tissue)

	Normal control group	Untreated diabetic group	Metformin treated group	L-Cysteine treated group	Combination treated group
N	10	10	10	10	10
X	9.12 [a]	24.76 [b]	18.69 [c]	15.44 [d]	12.78 [e]
S.D.	1.18	1.80	1.16	0.63	1.03
S.E.	0.37	0.57	0.37	0.20	0.33
F			239.031*		
p value			<0.001		
LSD			1.403		

X: Arithmetic mean   N: Number of animals
F: F test (ANOVA)
Different superscripts within each raw indicate statistically significant differences between groups at $p < 0.001$
* : Statistically significant at $p \leq 0.001$

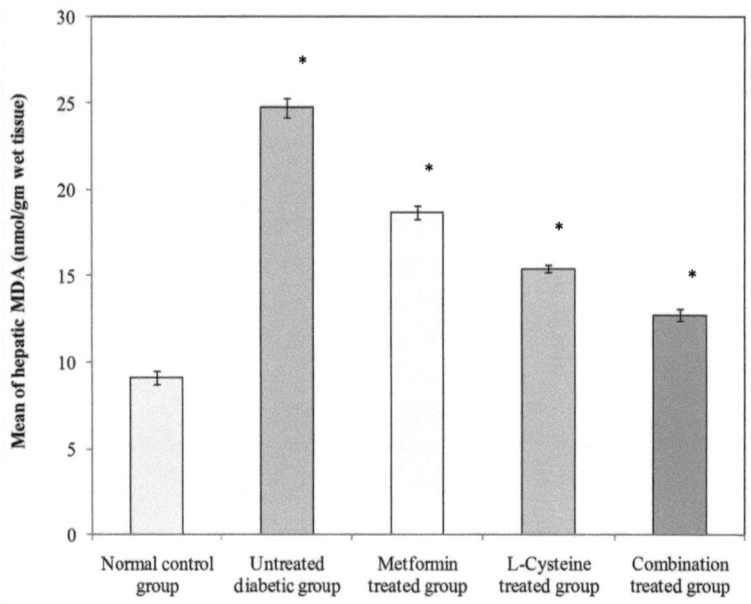

Figure (34): Effect of treatment with the studied drugs for 2 weeks on hepatic malondialdehyde in male albino rats

* : Significant in comparison to normal rats

3.2. Hepatic reduced glutathione (GSH)

• Metformin treated group

Treatment with metformin in a dose of 300 mg/kg/day for 2 weeks orally increased significantly the hepatic GSH mean level to reach a value of (171.35±1.56 µg/mg protein) versus (135.31±1.64 µg/mg protein) in the untreated diabetic rats at $p< 0.001$, (LSD $\geq$ 5.718). (Table 16) and (Figure 35)

• L-cysteine treated group

There was a significant increase in the hepatic GSH in the group treated with L-cysteine in a dose of 300 mg/kg/day for 2 weeks orally in comparison to the untreated diabetic rats at $p< 0.001$. The mean values of hepatic GSH for the two groups were (199.24±1.09 µg/mg protein) and (135.31±1.64 µg/mg protein) respectively, (LSD $\geq$ 5.718). (Table 16) and (Figure 35)

• Combination treated group

The study revealed that the combination treatment of metformin (300 mg/kg/day) and L-cysteine (300 mg/kg/day) orally for 2 weeks was associated with a significant increase in the hepatic GSH levels to reach a mean value (228.01±0.82 µg/mg protein) in comparison to the untreated diabetic group, in which the mean value of hepatic GSH was (135.31±1.64 µg/mg protein) at $p< 0.001$, (LSD $\geq$ 5.718). (Table 16) and (Figure 35)

Thus, treatment with metformin significantly increased the GSH values by 26.6% above the untreated diabetic values. The GSH levels in the L-cysteine treated group reached significantly higher values, about 47.2% above that of untreated diabetic group. Moreover, in the combination treatment group, the GSH content was more greatly increased as compared to the metformin and the L-cysteine treated groups, reaching a concentration about 68.5% that of untreated diabetic rats.

Table (16): Effect of treatment with the studied drugs for 2 weeks on hepatic reduced glutathione in male albino rats (µg/mg protein)

	Normal control group	Untreated diabetic group	Metformin treated group	L-Cysteine treated group	Combination treated group
N	10	10	10	10	10
X	250.10 [a]	135.31 [b]	171.35 [c]	199.24 [d]	228.01 [e]
S.D.	7.30	5.20	4.93	3.44	2.59
S.E.	2.31	1.64	1.56	1.09	0.82
F			837.078*		
p value			<0.001		
LSD			5.718		

X: Arithmetic mean N: Number of animals
F: F test (ANOVA)
Different superscripts within each raw indicate statistically significant differences between groups at $p < 0.001$
* : Statistically significant at $p \leq 0.001$

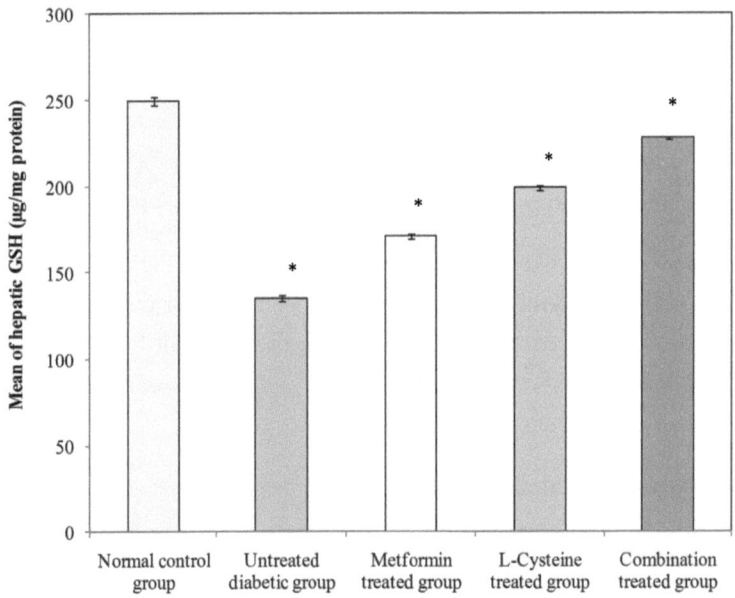

Figure (35): Effect of treatment with the studied drugs for 2 weeks on hepatic reduced glutathione in male albino rats

* : Significant in comparison to normal rats

4. Inflammatory parameters

4.1. Serum monocyte chemoattractant protein-1 (MCP-1)

- **Metformin treated group**

As could be seen in Table 17 and Figure 36, treatment of diabetic rats with metformin in a dose of 300 mg/kg/day for 2 weeks orally caused a significant decrease in serum level of MCP-1 (498.33±5.97 pg/ml) as compared to the mean value of untreated STZ-diabetic rats (670.42±9.01 pg/ml) at $p< 0.001$, (LSD $\geq$ 20.552).

- **L-cysteine treated group**

There was a significant decrease in serum MCP-1 in diabetic rats treated with L-cysteine in the aforementioned dose in comparison to the untreated diabetic rats at $p< 0.001$. The mean values for both groups were (369.70±4.87 pg/ml) and (670.42±9.01 pg/ml) respectively, (LSD $\geq$ 20.552). (Table 17) and (Figure 36)

- **Combination treated group**

It was also observed that the diabetic rats received metformin (300 mg/kg/day) and L-cysteine (300 mg/kg/day) orally in combination for 2 weeks showed a significant decrease in MCP-1 level in comparison to the untreated diabetic rats with mean values of (249.97±3.44 pg/ml) and (670.42±9.01 pg/ml) respectively at $p< 0.001$, (LSD $\geq$ 20.525). (Table 17) and (Figure 36)

Therefore, treatment with metformin for 2 weeks significantly decreased the MCP-1 values to an average of 25.7% below diabetic values. Oral L-cysteine treatment gave significantly lower levels of MCP-1 as compared to the metformin treated group, $p< 0.001$; reaching values lower than control diabetic values by about 44.9%. Combining both drugs together caused further significant reduction in the mean MCP-1 values to about 62.7% from STZ-diabetic levels.

Table (17): Effect of treatment with the studied drugs for 2 weeks on serum monocyte chemoattractant protein-1 in male albino rats (pg/ml)

	Normal control group	Untreated diabetic group	Metformin treated group	L-Cysteine treated group	Combination treated group
N	10	10	10	10	10
X	157.84 [a]	670.42 [b]	498.33 [c]	369.70 [d]	249.97 [e]
S.D.	8.22	28.49	18.87	15.40	10.88
S.E.	2.60	9.01	5.97	4.87	3.44
F			1290.550*		
p value			<0.001		
LSD			20.552		

X: Arithmetic mean N: Number of animals
F: F test (ANOVA)
Different superscripts within each raw indicate statistically significant differences between groups at $p < 0.001$
* : Statistically significant at $p \leq 0.001$

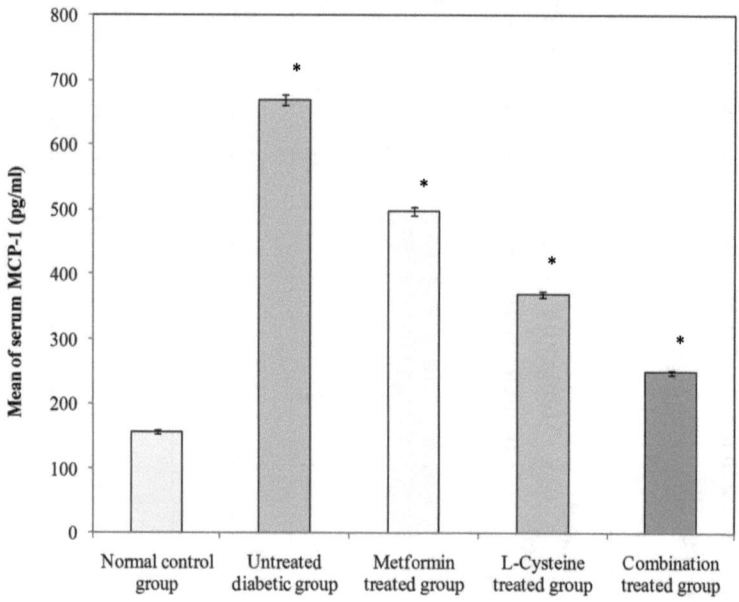

Figure (36): Effect of treatment with the studied drugs for 2 weeks on serum monocyte chemoattractant protein-1 in male albino rats

* : Significant in comparison to normal rats

4.2. Serum C-reactive protein (CRP)

- **Metformin treated group**

Treatment of STZ-diabetic rats with metformin in a dose of 300 mg/kg/day for 2 weeks orally caused a significant reduction in the mean value of CRP to reach a value of (2.27±0.07 mg/L) when compared to the untreated diabetic rats with mean value (3.25±0.08 mg/L) at p< 0.001, (LSD ≥ 0.229). (Table 18) and (Figure 37)

- **L-cysteine treated group**

A significant decrease in serum CRP was observed in the diabetic rats treated with L-cysteine, in a dose of 300 mg/kg/day given orally for 2 weeks, in comparison to the untreated diabetic rats at p< 0.001. The mean values of serum CRP were (1.54±0.06 mg/L) and (3.25±0.08 mg/L) respectively, (LSD ≥ 0.229). (Table 18) and (Figure 37)

- **Combination treated group**

Treating STZ-diabetic rats with both oral metformin in a dose of 300 mg/kg/day and oral L-cysteine in a dose of 300 mg/kg/day for 2 weeks resulted in a significant decrease in serum CRP as compared to the untreated diabetic rats at p< 0.001. The mean value of serum CRP was decreased from (3.25±0.08 mg/L) in the untreated STZ-diabetic group to (0.88±0.06 mg/L) after treatment with both drugs in combination, (LSD ≥ 0.229), (Table 18) and (Figure 37).

Similarly, the effect of L-cysteine was more substantial than that of metformin on the serum CRP level. Both metformin and L-cysteine caused significant decreases in CRP levels, reaching values about 30.2% and 52.6% lower than the untreated diabetic values. In the combination treatment group, the effect on CRP was more profound as the level went down by approximately 73% from the untreated diabetic values. All decreases carried a statistical significance of p< 0.001.

Table (18): Effect of treatment with the studied drugs for 2 weeks on serum C-reactive protein in male albino rats (mg/L)

	Normal control group	Untreated diabetic group	Metformin treated group	L-Cysteine treated group	Combination treated group
N	10	10	10	10	10
X	0.40 [a]	3.25 [b]	2.27 [c]	1.54 [d]	0.88 [e]
S.D.	0.09	0.27	0.23	0.19	0.18
S.E.	0.03	0.08	0.07	0.06	0.06
F			323.444*		
p value			<0.001		
LSD			0.229		

X: Arithmetic mean   N: Number of animals
F: F test (ANOVA)
Different superscripts within each raw indicate statistically significant differences between groups at $p < 0.001$
* : Statistically significant at $p \leq 0.001$

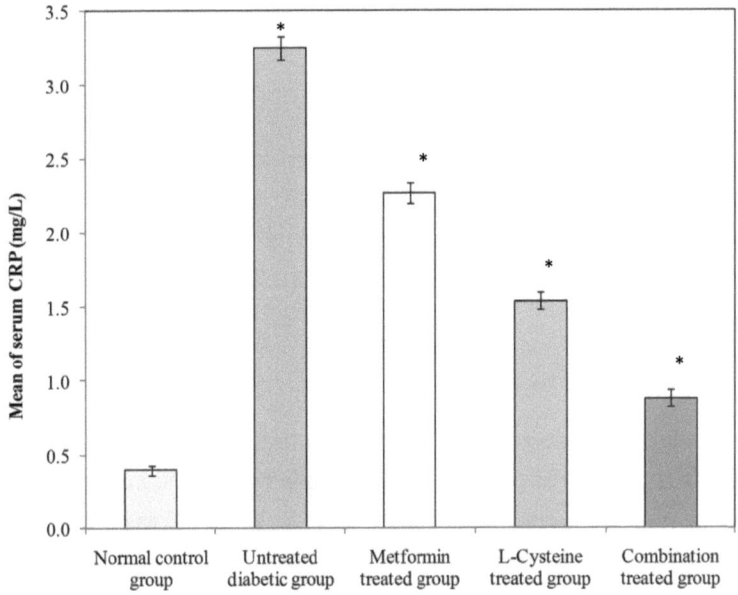

Figure (37): Effect of treatment with the studied drugs for 2 weeks on serum C-reactive protein in male albino rats

* : Significant in comparison to normal rats

4.3. Serum nitric oxide (NO)

- **Metformin treated group**

STZ-diabetic rats treated with metformin in a dose of 300 mg/kg/day for 2 weeks orally showed a significant decrease in the serum NO level to reach a mean value of (37.04±0.94 nmol/ml) in comparison to the mean value of the untreated diabetic rats, which was (65.95±2.07 nmol/ml) at $p<0.001$, (LSD ≥ 4.032). (Table 19) and (Figure 38)

- **L-cysteine treated group**

There was a significant reduction in serum NO from its mean value in the untreated STZ-diabetic group (65.95±2.07 nmol/ml) to reach a value of (46.51±0.54 nmol/ml) in the group treated with L-cysteine in a dose of 300 mg/kg/day for 2 week orally at $p<0.001$, (LSD ≥ 4.032). (Table 19) and (Figure 38)

- **Combination treated group**

A significant decrease was resulted in the mean value of serum NO in STZ-diabetic rats treated with combination between both metformin and L-cysteine, in the aforementioned dose for 2 weeks orally, as compared to the untreated diabetic rats at $p<0.001$. The mean values for the two groups were (27.01±0.51 nmol/ml) and (65.95±2.07 nmol/ml) respectively, (LSD ≥ 4.032). (Table 19) and (Figure 38)

In contrast to L-cysteine's stronger effect on MCP-1 and CRP, it caused a smaller reduction in NO levels as compared to the metformin treated group. Nitric oxide values averaged 70.5% and 56.2% of the untreated diabetic values in the L-cysteine and metformin treated groups respectively, $p<0.001$. Greater reductions in nitric oxide levels were observed in the combination treatment group reaching values about 59% below the STZ-diabetic levels, $p<0.001$.

Table (19): Effect of treatment with the studied drugs for 2 weeks on serum nitric oxide in male albino rats (nmol/ml)

	Normal control group	Untreated diabetic group	Metformin treated group	L-Cysteine treated group	Combination treated group
N	10	10	10	10	10
X	18.77 [a]	65.95 [b]	37.04 [c]	46.51 [d]	27.01 [e]
S.D.	1.96	6.56	2.98	1.71	1.62
S.E.	0.62	2.07	0.94	0.54	0.51
F			273.426*		
p value			<0.001		
LSD			4.032		

X: Arithmetic mean N: Number of animals
F: F test (ANOVA)
Different superscripts within each raw indicate statistically significant differences between groups at $p < 0.001$
* : Statistically significant at $p \leq 0.001$

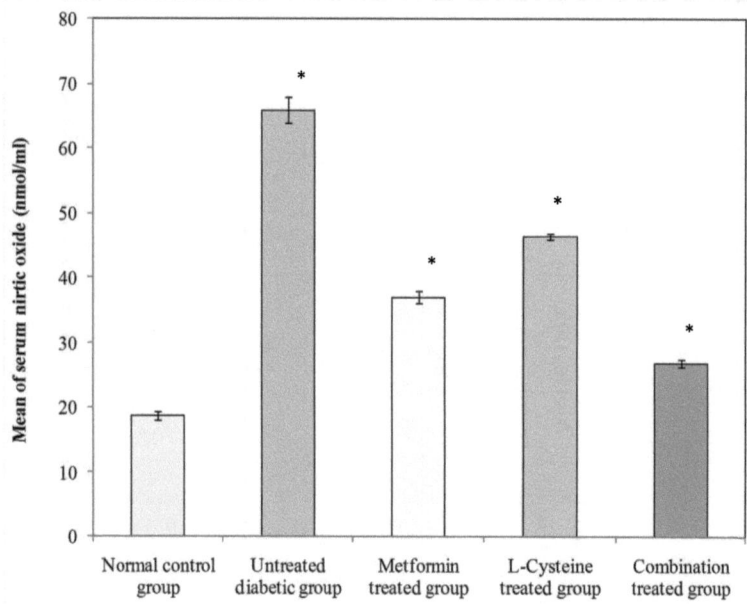

Figure (38): Effect of treatment with the studied drugs for 2 weeks on serum nitric oxide in male albino rats

* : Significant in comparison to normal rats

5. Histopathological examination of pancreas

Pancreatic islet cells from control rats exhibited normal architecture, namely normal size and shape with eosinophilic cytoplasm and centrally placed nuclei (Fig. 39A). Degenerated islets with irregular contour, cytoplasmic vacuolization and apoptotic cells were observed in pancreatic tissue from untreated diabetic rats (Fig. 39B). Treatment of diabetic rats with either L-cysteine (Fig. 39C) or metformin (Fig. 39D) resulted in moderate regeneration of pancreatic islets. Well formed regenerating islets were observed in rats treated with both drugs in combination (Fig. 39E) indicating more protection against pancreatic tissue damage.

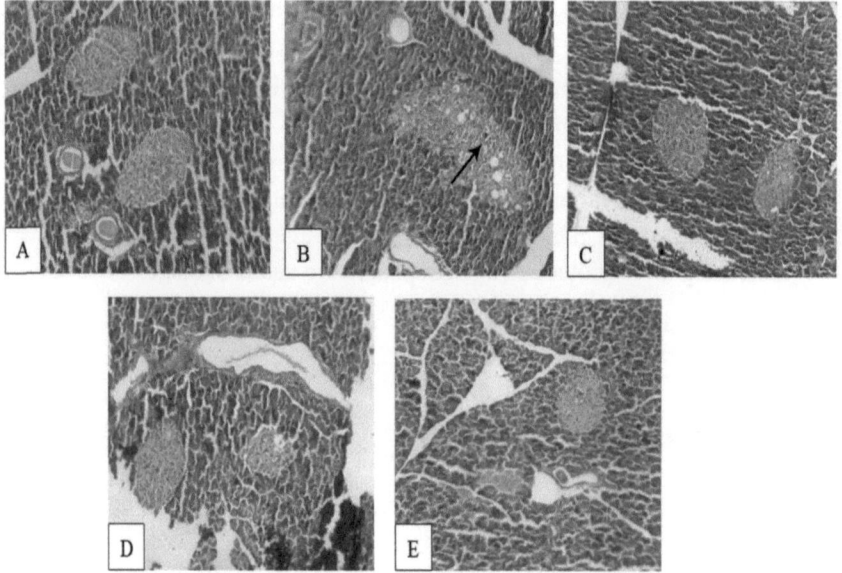

Figure (39): Histopathological evaluation of pancreatic sections stained with hematoxylin and eosin (H&E) stain (X 10).

(A) Section of normal pancreas showing pancreatic islets of normal size and shape with centrally placed nuclei.

(B) Pancreatic section of diabetic rats showing degenerated islet of irregular shape with cytoplasmic vacuolization and apoptotic cells (indicated by arrow).

(C & D) Pancreatic sections of L-cysteine-treated and metformin-treated rats respectively, showing moderately regenerating islets.

(E) Section of the pancreas of the combined therapy group showing well formed regenerated islet.

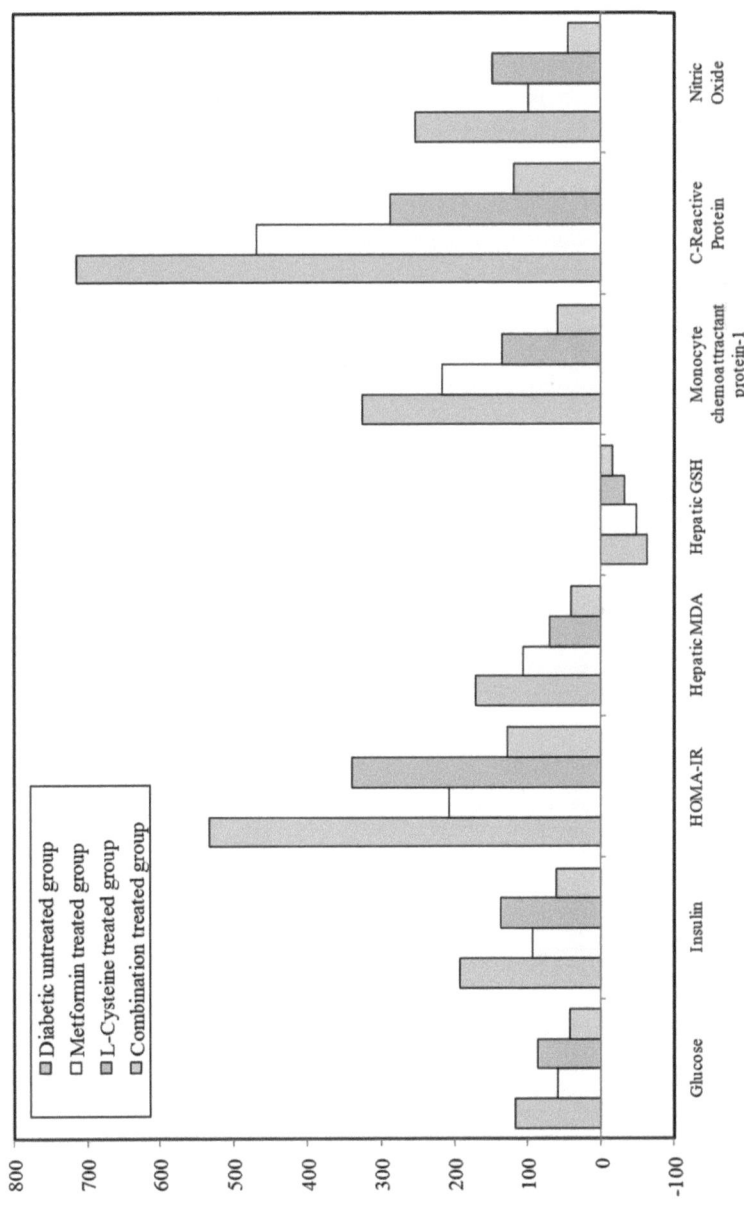

Figure (40): Comparison of mean percentage change in biochemical metabolic, oxidative stress and inflammatory parameters between untreated and treated (metformin, L-cysteine and their combination) experimentally induced type 2 diabetic adult male rats

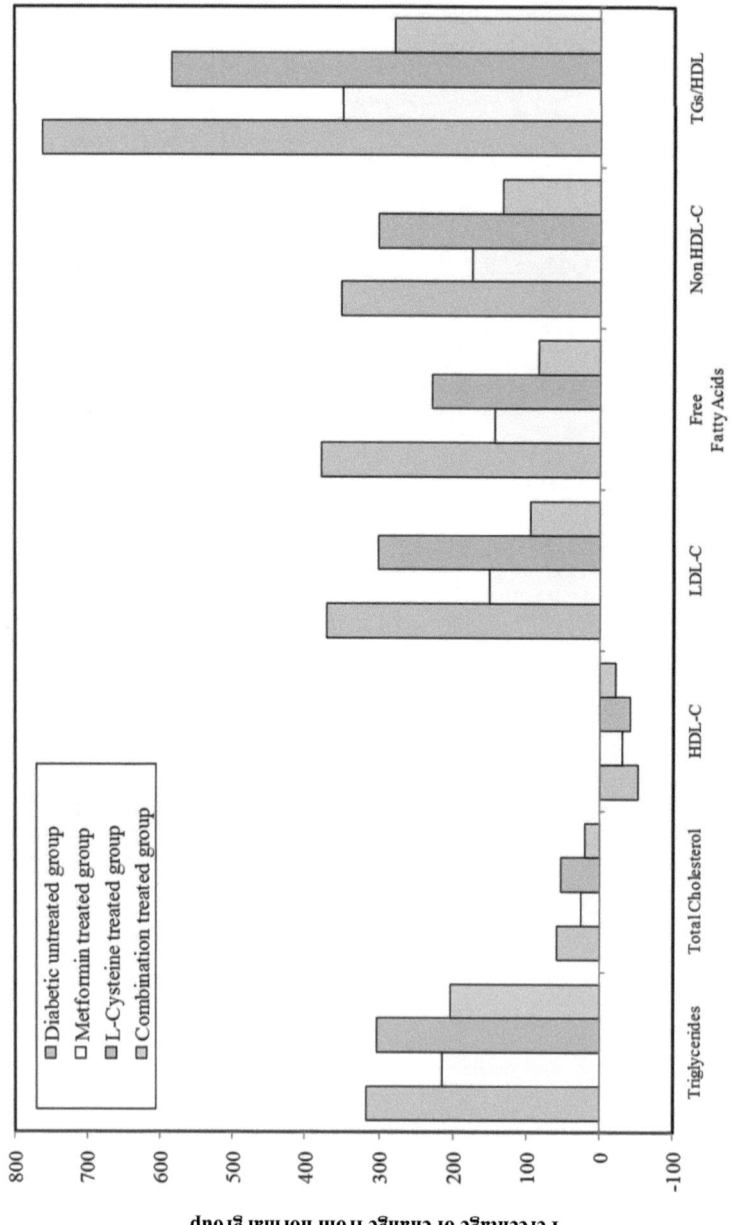

Figure (41): Comparison of mean percentage change in lipid profile between untreated and treated (metformin, L-cysteine and their combination) experimentally induced type 2 diabetic adult male rats

DISCUSSION

Diabetes mellitus is a multifactorial metabolic syndrome, affecting at least 150 million people worldwide and causing many serious socio-economic problems. It is characterized by absolute or relative deficiency of insulin and pancreatic polypeptide secretion and imperfection of insulin receptor or post-receptor events with derangement in carbohydrate, protein and lipid metabolism. Insulin resistance is the core pathophysiological feature in type 2 diabetes mellitus, leading to increased hepatic glucose production and decreased glucose uptake and disposal. This is followed by decreased insulin secretion, as a result of progressive pancreatic β-cell dysfunction. These dual defects eventually result in chronic hyperglycemia, a clinical hallmark of diabetes mellitus [257-259].

Indeed, chronic hyperglycemia is contemplated to produce a notable decline in the level of intracellular antioxidants and to generate proxidants through diverse pathways. These pathways include mutilation of the redox equilibrium, augmentation of advanced glycation products, glycosylation of antioxidative enzymes, activation of protein kinase C or overproduction of mitochondrial superoxides. These finally lead to oxidative stress in various tissues [257], particularly in pancreatic β-cells, which are highly susceptible to damage by ROS due to low antioxidant enzymes expression [260]. In type 2 diabetes, ROS activate β-cell apoptotic pathways, impair insulin synthesis and also contribute to insulin resistance and diabetic complications [261].

Nowadays, increasing evidence from human population studies and animal research has established correlative as well as causative links between chronic inflammation and insulin resistance, which leads finally to type 2 diabetes mellitus [262]. There is now a wealth of evidence, indicating close ties between metabolic and immune systems from an emerging paradigm that metabolic imbalance; with starvation and immunosuppression on one end of the spectrum and obesity and inflammatory diseases on the other end [263].

Obesity, particularly visceral obesity, and its associated hyperlipidemia are hallmarks and major risk factors of type 2 diabetes mellitus. Adipose tissue plays an important role in the development of inflammation, insulin resistance and type 2 diabetes mellitus. Resistance of dysfunctional fat cells to the antilipolytic effects of insulin leads to chronic elevation in plasma FFAs levels. These cells, in turn, produce excessive amounts of cytokines such as TNF-α, IL-6 and resistin that further increase insulin resistance, inflammation and atherosclerosis, as well as, these cells secrete reduced amounts of insulin sensitizing cytokines such as adiponectin [264]. Moreover, elevated circulating levels of FFAs, which are derived from adipocytes, contribute to insulin resistance by inhibiting glucose uptake, glycogen synthesis and glycolysis, as well as by increasing hepatic glucose production [265]. FFAs were reported to stimulate expression of gluconeogenic enzymes, including glucose-6-phosphatase [266].

Although the antidiabetic drugs may be effective for glycemic control in type 2 diabetes mellitus, at least in the early stages, they do not appear to be effective in entirely preventing the progression of ROS-mediated organ damage [261]. The pathophysiological changes in type 2 diabetes mellitus sets the scene for considering antioxidant and anti-inflammatory therapy, together with reduction in visceral adiposity and tissue lipid content, as an adjunct to the commonly used oral antidiabetics in the management of this disease [1]. There are several available antioxidants that hold promise as new approaches for the treatment of insulin resistance and type 2 diabetes mellitus, including N-acetyl cysteine and α-lipoic acid [149].

Therefore, the aim of the present study was to investigate the metabolic derangements, dyslipidemia, oxidative stress and inflammation associated with experimentally-induced type 2 diabetes mellitus. Moreover, it was conducted to evaluate the metabolic and lipid profile improvements as well as the antioxidant and anti-inflammatory effects of the amino acid, L-cysteine in the management of STZ-induced rat model of type 2 DM. The study was also designed to assess any possible additive effect of L-cysteine with the well-established gold star antidiabetic drug, metformin, on the aforementioned parameters in the STZ-induced type 2 diabetes in rats.

For induction of a rat model of type 2 diabetes, rats were initially fed with high fat diet, which was used to produce insulin resistance, an early feature of type 2 diabetes. This is followed by injecting rats with a low dose of streptozotocin, which has been known to induce a mild impairment of insulin secretion. Therefore, this rat model closely mimics the natural history of the disease events, which progresses from insulin resistance to β-cells dysfunction as well as resembles metabolic characteristics of type 2 diabetes in human [267].

The results of the present study revealed that injecting rats with a low dose of streptozotocin after their maintenance on high fat diet for 2 months was associated with hyperglycemia, hyperinsulinemia and insulin resistance, which was presented by calculating HOMA-IR, a mathematical model that relates fasting glucose and insulin levels to insulin resistance. These findings were in accordance with the results, previously reported by Zhang et al in 2003 [237] and Abdin et al in 2010 [39].

High fat diet (HFD) has been shown to induce insulin resistance by different mechanisms, but considered mainly through Randle or glucose-fatty acid cycle. Briefly, the presence of high level of triglycerides due to excess fat intake could constitute a source of increased fatty acid availability and oxidation. The preferential use of increased fatty acids for oxidation blunts the insulin-mediated reduction of hepatic glucose output and reduces the glucose uptake and utilization in skeletal muscle leading to compensatory hyperinsulinemia, a common feature of insulin resistance [268]. This explains the hyperinsulinemia observed in our animal model. Another potential mechanism of high fat diet-induced insulin resistance could involve the activation of PKC and inhibitor of NF-κB kinase-β (IKKβ) by the elevated FFAs level. These serine kinases are mediators of inflammation, resulting in the inhibition of insulin-stimulated glucose transport [149]. FFAs also affect insulin-signaling pathway where their elevated levels impair IRS-1 phosphorylation and PI3K activation following insulin stimulation [269].

Conversion of this insulin resistant state to overt type 2 diabetes with frank hyperglycemia was achieved by the low dose streptozotocin. STZ induces β-cell death through DNA alkylation and increasing the β-cells oxidative stress thus establishing a state of relative insulin deficiency and hyperglycemia [267]. Elevation of blood glucose may be attributed to reduced entry of glucose to peripheral tissues, muscle and adipose tissue, increased glycogen breakdown and increased gluconeogenesis [270].

Moreover, the results of the present study revealed that STZ-induced diabetic rats showed significant increases in serum triglycerides, total cholesterol, LDL-C, free fatty acids, calculated non-HDL-cholesterol and triglycerides to HDL-C ratio, in addition to a significant decrease in serum HDL-C level.

In agreement to our results, a previous study reported that the levels of triglycerides and total cholesterol were further accentuated after STZ injection to high fat diet-fed rats[268]. Sahin et al in 2007 [271] also showed that high fat diet and STZ induced type 2 diabetic rats were hypertriglyceridemic and hypercholesterolemic. Another recent study reported that type 2 diabetes in rats induced by HFD and low dose STZ was associated with significant increases in serum levels of triglycerides, total cholesterol, LDL-C and FFAs as well as a significant decrease in HDL-C [272].

In addition, many studies in the literature showed the characteristic atherogenic dyslipidemia associated with diabetes in both diabetic animals and humans, which was seen as increased levels of triglycerides, total cholesterol, LDL-C, non-HDL-cholesterol and free fatty acids as well as reduced HDL-C [273-275].

Hypertriglyceridemia may be caused by the increased hepatic TGs production or decreased TGs removal or both. In insulin resistant states, lipolysis is stimulated in adipose tissues, increasing the delivery of FFAs from adipose tissues to liver and consequently increases the hepatic lipid content and circulating TGs-rich VLDL production. Moreover, hyperinsulinemia enhances the expression of hepatic sterol regulatory element binding protein (SREBP), a key transcription factor. SREBP can activate a cascade of enzymes involved in fatty acid and cholesterol biosynthesis, such as fatty acid synthase (FAS) and HMG-CoA reductase[276]. Since liver TGs production is mainly determined by the free fatty acid synthesis rate, which is controlled at the level of transcription by SREBP, thus induction of SREBP expression will finally result in a rise in triglycerides [277]. Hypertriglyceridemia may be also due to a defect in lipoprotein lipase, which hydrolyzes circulating TGs, causing impaired plasma triglyceride removal. In addition, it was reported that STZ-diabetic rats exhibited VLDL receptor deficiency in skeletal muscle, heart and adipose tissue thus decreasing VLDL clearance[278].

Therefore, the hypertriglyceridemia observed in our rat model of type 2 diabetes may be due to increased absorption and formation of triglycerides in the form of chylomicrons following exogenous consumption of diet rich in fat or through increased endogenous production of TGs-enriched hepatic very low-density lipoprotein (VLDL) and decreased TGs uptake in peripheral tissue [268].

The increase in total cholesterol and LDL-C demonstrated in our results was in accordance to a previous study, which showed that serum total cholesterol and LDL-C levels were elevated in a model of STZ-induced type 2 diabetes in rats [279]. It was also showed in another recent study that hyperglycemia was accompanied with a marked increase in total cholesterol, LDL-C and triglycerides as well as a reduction in HDL-C in HFD/STZ diabetic rats [270].

Serum cholesterol levels are mainly incorporated in LDL fraction, indicating harmful effects. This frank hypercholesterolemia, found in our rat model of type 2 diabetes mellitus, may be attributed to increased dietary cholesterol absorption from the small intestine following the intake of high fat diet [268] or may be due to increased rate of cholesterol synthesis which is stimulated 2-3 fold in the gut of STZ-induced diabetic rats [280]. Furthermore, increases in VLDL secretion can lead to chain reactions in other lipoprotein and lipids, leading to the increased levels of LDL-C and total cholesterol[276]. It was also reported that the status of hyperglycemia can accelerate LDL modifications with subsequent AGEs formation [281].

Moreover, insulin resistant and diabetic states are associated with a reduction in HDL-C, which is one of the main defenses against atherosclerosis. Beside its role in reverse cholesterol transport, HDL has an array of antioxidant mechanisms which may prevent the formation and promote removal of lipid peroxides from cell membranes and from other lipoproteins such as the proatherogenic LDL [282].

Our study revealed a decrease in serum HDL-C. This was in accordance to a previous study which showed dyslipidemia with a significant decrease in HDL-C level in STZ-induced diabetic rats [283]. This decrease in circulating HDL seen in insulin resistant states is intimately linked to the overproduction of TGs-rich lipoproteins such as VLDL and chylomicrons. Although the mechanisms are not entirely clear, available data implicate TGs-enrichment of HDL particles leading to particle instability and degradation. The interaction between HDL that is TGs enriched and hepatic lipase action has been suggested to play an important role in the enhanced catabolism of HDL in insulin resistant, hypertriglyceridemic states [276].

Our results also showed an elevated fasting serum FFAs. This was in accordance to previous studies which showed a significant elevation in the concentration of FFAs in high fat diet/STZ diabetic rats [39, 271]. The net plasma concentration of FFAs results from a delicate equilibrium between enzyme-regulated lipolysis of plasma triglycerides-rich lipoproteins such as VLDL, lipolysis of TGs stored in adipose tissue and FFAs uptake by peripheral tissues. Under normal conditions, insulin stimulates postprandial uptake of glucose, as well as FFAs esterification and storage. Insulin and glucose are also believed to regulate lipoprotein lipase (LPL) activity, which provides an essential first step in the delivery of FFAs to adipose tissue for storage, as well as plasma TGs removal. In the insulin resistant state, there is an increase in release of FFAs from adipose tissue. This may result in an increased influx of FFAs into the liver and the muscle. This "vicious cycle" may result in attenuation in insulin signaling in these tissues and may exacerbate insulin resistance [276]. Thus increased free fatty acids flux from adipose tissue to non-adipose tissues resulting from abnormalities in fat metabolism; either in storage or lipolysis, is both a consequence of insulin resistance and aggravating factor, participating in and amplifying many of the fundamental metabolic derangements that are characteristic to insulin resistance and type 2 diabetes [284].

In our research, a significant elevation in the levels of the calculated atherogenic indices, non-HDL-cholesterol and triglycerides to HDL-C ratio, was observed. These two indices are particularly useful in predicting cardiovascular disease risk in patients with diabetes [285, 286]. High TGs/HDL-C ratio was also reported to correlate with the small dense LDL and insulin resistance [286].

Furthermore, the results of the present study revealed a significant increase in hepatic malondialdehyde concentration and a significant decrease in hepatic reduced glutathione content in the high fat diet/STZ induced type 2 diabetes in rats.

These results indicate the presence of oxidative stress with subsequent cellular damage in the liver of STZ-induced rat model of type 2 diabetes mellitus. Oxidative stress with excessive generation of free radicals and depleted levels of free radical scavenging enzymes have been demonstrated in both experimental animal models of diabetes and human diabetic subjects. Oxygen radicals are the major causative agents for distant organ damage as increased production of $OH^{\cdot}$, $O_2^{\cdot-}$ and H_2O_2 have detrimental effects on various tissues. Our findings were in accordance to previous studies which showed that high fat diet/STZ type 2 diabetic rats had a significant elevation in hepatic MDA concentrations [271, 287]. An earlier study also reported a significant increase in the MDA level, which was due to decreased activity of most of the antioxidant enzymes [288]. This increase in MDA was correlated with hyperglycemia in diabetic patients [289]. Furthermore, previous studies showed a significant reduction in the level of reduced glutathione in liver and serum of HFD/STZ diabetic rats [287, 290]. In addition, many studies showed a marked decreased level of reduced glutathione in the plasma of diabetic patients [79, 291, 292].

Increased oxidant production and subsequent antioxidants consumption in diabetic and insulin-resistant states can originate from the metabolism of both glucose and FFAs[293]. Abundant evidences demonstrate that chronic exposure to high circulating glucose or FFAs increases ROS production, that in turn causes lipid peroxidation and membrane damage, as well as decreases insulin content and glucose-stimulated insulin secretion of β-cells [68]. Lipid peroxidation provides useful information for prognosis of diabetes. It is frequently used as an index of tissue oxidative stress, in which oxygen interacts with polyunsaturated fatty acids and leads to the formation of toxic products such as MDA that plays an important role in the pathogenesis and progression of diabetes and its complications [290].

Increased ROS production results from hyperglycemia-induced increase in the proton gradient across the inner mitochondrial membrane. When the gradient exceeds a threshold, complex III electron transfer is blocked, leading to leakage of electrons, with formation of superoxide [294]. This increased superoxide production is the central and major mediator of diabetes tissue damage. [295]. It is hypothesized that excess ROS inhibits the glycolytic enzyme, glyceraldehyde-3-phosphate dehydrogenase. This inhibition in turn mediates the activation of the proposed mechanisms of hyperglycemia-associated tissue damage [294] and leads to direct inactivation of eNOS as well as results in decreases in insulin promoter activity, insulin gene transcription and expression, insulin secretion, induction of β-cells apoptosis and impairment in energy production, contributing to the development and progression of diabetes mellitus [57].

Hyperglycemia also results in increased flux through the polyol pathway causing NADPH depletion, impaired glutathione reductase activity and a decrease in the GSH:GSSG ratio. In addition, increased AGEs formation and their binding to RAGE receptors result in generating more ROS, increasing GPx activity and depleting of glutathione; which may further enhance lipid peroxidation [296]. Moreover, elevated FFAs have numerous adverse effects on mitochondrial function, including the uncoupling of oxidative phosphorylation and generation of more ROS, including superoxide, thus impairing endogenous antioxidant defenses by reducing intracellular glutathione [297]. This depletion of GSH leads to hamper the stabilizing effects of GSH on NO. Thus, in diabetes, excessive formation of superoxide anion ($O_2^{\cdot -}$) resulted which in turn, by a direct reaction with nitric oxide (NO), results in the formation of peroxynitrite (ONOO$^-$), a potent oxidant. ONOO$^-$ was found to be strongly correlated with oxidative stress and apoptosis. However, under physiological conditions, $O_2^{\cdot -}$ is predominantly removed by SOD and the formation of ONOO$^-$ will be minimal [298].

The results of the present study revealed that high fat diet/STZ diabetic rats showed a significant increase in the serum levels of the inflammatory markers; monocyte chemoattractant protein-1 (MCP-1), C-reactive protein (CRP) and nitric oxide (NO).

Our results were in accordance to a previous study which showed significant increased levels of TNF-α, IL-6 and CRP, which were all in significant positive correlation with insulin resistance (HOMA-IR) in the diabetic experimental rat model [39]. It was also reported that the inflammatory marker; CRP, a non-specific acute phase reactant, is commonly elevated in human insulin resistant states [299]. Moreover, it was reported that animal models of obesity have shown significant increases in circulating proinflammatory mediators including CRP, MCP-1 and IL-6 [300]. In addition, a recent study showed a significant increase in the level of MCP-1 in an animal model of type 2 diabetes; Goto-Kakizaki rats fed with high fat diet [301]. A previous study showed also a significant increase in the serum nitric oxide level in STZ diabetic rats fed with fat containing diet [302]. However, another study reported a decrease in the serum level of NO in the HFD/STZ type 2 diabetic rats [303]. The reasons for these discrepancies between our results and them are not clear, but may be related to the different animal models, different STZ dose used, severity and time course of hyperglycemia.

Inflammation is strongly suggested as a primary cause of obesity-linked insulin resistance, hyperglycemia, hyperlipidemia and atherosclerosis rather than merely a consequence [263]. Nowadays, the circulating inflammatory markers and the acute phase reactants are considered strong predictors for the development of type 2 diabetes and its possible associated cardiovascular complications [304].

The inhibition of signaling downstream of the insulin receptor is a primary mechanism through which inflammatory signaling leads to insulin resistance. This was assured by exposure of cells to TNF-α which stimulates inhibitory phosphorylation of serine residues of IRS-1. This phosphorylation reduces both tyrosine phosphorylation of IRS-1 and its ability to associate with the insulin receptor and thereby inhibits downstream signaling and insulin action, decreasing insulin sensitivity [70, 263]. This might, in turn, interfere with the anti-inflammatory effect of insulin, promoting further inflammation. It was reported that a low dose infusion of insulin suppresses intranuclear NF-κB binding and reduces plasma intercellular adhesion molecule-1 (ICAM-1), plasma tissue factor, PAI-1 and monocyte chemotactic protein-1 (MCP-1) concentrations. An interruption of insulin signal transduction would prevent the anti-inflammatory effect of insulin from being exerted [305].

Moreover, it was found that the expression of multiple genes in vascular cells, including redox-sensitive transcription factors (such as NF-κB) could be activated by oxidative stress. Overexpression of these genes stimulates the secretion of many proinflammatory cytokines such as TNF-α, IL-6 and MCP-1. The increasing level of these markers is known to decrease insulin sensitivity and increase vascular inflammation. Thus, oxidative stress plays a key role in the regulatory pathway that progresses from elevated glucose to monocyte and endothelial cell activation in the enhanced vascular inflammation of diabetes [75]. It was reported that in hyperglycemic conditions, the increased glucose uptake by endothelial cells causes excess production of ROS in mitochondria, which inflicts oxidative damage and activates inflammatory signaling cascades, resulting in endothelial injury that in turn might attract inflammatory cells such as macrophages and further exacerbate the local inflammation [70]. This can be explained by the findings of a previously published study showed that transient exposure of cultured human aortic endothelial to hyperglycemia induces persistent epigenetic changes in the promoter of the NF-κB, leading to a sustained increase in the expression of the NF-κB responsive proatherogenic genes MCP-1 and VCAM-1 as well as the proinflammatory genes, IL-6 and iNOS [306].

The plasma level of C-reactive protein was found to be increased in both T1DM and T2DM. It plays a significant role in inflammation and atherogenesis. CRP causes numerous proinflammatory and proatherogenic effects in endothelial cells, such as decreased endothelial NO and prostacyclin and increased cell adhesion molecules; MCP-1, IL-8 and PAI-1 [307]. In monocytes/macrophages, CRP increases ROS and proinflammatory cytokine release, promotes monocyte chemotaxis and adhesion and increases oxidized LDL uptake. Moreover, in vascular smooth muscle cells, CRP has been shown to increase inducible NO production and increase NF-κB activity, resulting in increased oxidative stress and vascular smooth muscle cell proliferation [308].

Monocyte chemoattractant protein-1 (MCP-1, also known as chemokine ligand 2 (Ccl2)) and its cognate receptor chemokine receptor 2 (Ccr2) are also major components of insulin resistance [299]. MCP-1 plays important roles in the vascular inflammatory process through its multiple actions, which include recruitment of neutrophils and T lymphocytes into the subendothelial space, monocyte adhesion to endothelium and migration of vascular smooth muscle cells [73]. Many studies on the MCP-1have shown that its expression is increased in obese mice, suggesting that changes in its level promote the recruitment of macrophages to adipose tissue and cause inhibition of tyrosine phosphorylation in liver and skeletal muscle, resulting in inflammation and insulin resistance [73, 74, 299].

A very important mediator synthesized by endothelial cells is nitric oxide (NO), because of its vasodilatory, antiplatelet, antiproliferative, anti-inflammatory and antioxidant properties. NO inhibits adhesion of leucocytes as well as cytokine-induced expression of vascular cell adhesion molecule-1 (VCAM-1) and monocyte chemotactic protein-1 (MCP-1), probably through the inhibition of the transcription factor nuclear factor-κB[307]. NO is rapidly inactivated by $O_2^{.-}$, a major potential pathway of NO reactivity. Oxidative breakdown of NO gives rise to radicals such as peroxynitrite and peroxynitrous acid, not only decreasing NO levels but increasing oxidative stress [115].

The endothelium of diabetic subjects is a great producer of superoxide instead of NO[309], resulting in a decreased NO/ROS ratio. This undesirable effect may be due to endothelial nitric oxide synthase (eNOS) uncoupling, which results from many factors. These include the oxidative stress as eNOS contains a free cysteine SH group at its catalytic site, making it susceptible to inactivation by ROS and aldehydes [115], as well as the increased production of nitroarginine, a competitive inhibitor for L-arginine, the substrate for generating NO [309].

Several inducers of insulin resistance, including FFAs, proinflammatory cytokines and oxidative stress, activate the expression of NOS-2, the gene that encodes iNOS, a mediator of non-specific tissue damage leading to excessive nitric oxide production [299, 310]. It was reported that iNOS induction is associated with impaired insulin action in skeletal muscle, indicating that iNOS may be involved in the pathogenesis of chronic metabolic disorders such as atherosclerosis, insulin resistance and obesity-linked type 2 diabetes in which an inflammatory condition is believed to play a pathologic role [310]. In the insulin signaling pathway, NO can reduce Akt activity by causing s-nitrosylation of a specific cysteine residue. Increased iNOS activity also results in the degradation of IRS-1 in cultured skeletal muscle cells [299]. Moreover, overexpression of iNOS mRNA in the pancreatic islets of Zucker diabetic rats suggested that high NO production in this tissue might cause impaired insulin secretion [310]. On the other hand, eNOS expression decreases in the insulin resistance syndrome, triggering endothelial dysfunction [310], as it was showed that its level is partially regulated by insulin [115].

Nitric oxide and NO donors have been demonstrated to have an autoinhibition capacity of NOS via specific binding sites on the enzyme; however, a relatively marked lower concentration of NO is required for inhibition of constitutive NOS (eNOS and nNOS) than for iNOS. Therefore, it is possible that, in metabolic syndrome, insulin resistance and type 2 diabetes mellitus, the associated state of proatherogenesis and low-grade inflammation increases cytokines such as TNF-α and IL-1 levels, causing iNOS induction, producing a substantial concentrations of NO that could autoinhibit the cNOS in-vivo, resulting in a condition in which iNOS is overexpressed while cNOS is concurrently inhibited [310]. In our study, serum NO levels were higher in diabetic rats, supporting the hypothesis that NO overproduction in acute hyperglycemia may be associated with eNOS inhibition and iNOS overexpression.

As mentioned, type 2 diabetes is a complex progressive disorder that is difficult to treat effectively in the long-term. The majority of patients is obese at diagnosis and will be unable to achieve or sustain near normoglycemia without oral antidiabetic agent [183]. Metformin is the gold star in treatment of diabetes, whose history dates to medieval times. Metformin is currently the drug of first choice for the treatment of type 2 diabetes, being prescribed to at least 120 million people worldwide. Furthermore, metformin has been used against the development of type 2 DM in high-risk persons, with a 31% reduction in incidence [311]

In our present study, treatment of STZ-diabetic rats with metformin in a dose of 300 mg/kg/day for 2 weeks orally resulted in a significant decrease in the levels of fasting serum glucose, insulin and HOMA-IR as compared to the untreated diabetic rats.

These findings are in accordance to metformin's well known antihyperglycemic effects already described in both animals and human studies [312, 313]. However, we also showed in our research that the metformin treated group exhibited better metabolic control than L-cysteine group. This was also assured by HOMA-IR, which indicated that reduction in insulin resistance by metformin is significantly better than L-cysteine. This is probably secondary to the increased insulin sensitivity and concomitant decrease in hyperglycemia.

Metformin exerts an antihyperglycemic effect, primarily by suppressing basal hepatic glucose production mainly through inhibiting gluconeogenesis and by increasing glucose disposal in skeletal muscle [167]. This preferential action of metformin in hepatocytes is due to the predominant expression of organic cation transporter-1 (OCT1), which has been shown to facilitate cellular uptake of metformin [314]. Metformin also increases insulin sensitivity by 20–25%, mainly by promoting weight loss[149]. Although this effect on weight varies between patient populations, it is preferred for obese patients[167]. A recent study suggests that increased OCT1 gene expression in adipose tissue of obese subjects might contribute to the increased metformin action in these subjects [315].

A previous study reported that metformin treatment caused an increase in insulin sensitivity, resulted from significant increases in visfatin and adiponectin [316]. Although the function of visfatin is not currently understood, visfatin may have a dual role; an autocrine/paracrine function that facilitates differentiation and fat deposition on visceral adipose tissue and an endocrine role that modulate insulin sensitivity in peripheral organs[317].

The results of the present study also showed that treatment of STZ-diabetic rats with metformin in a dose of 300 mg/kg/day for 2 weeks orally was associated with significant improvements in lipid profile as compared to the untreated diabetic rats. This was revealed by significant decreases in serum triglycerides, total cholesterol, LDL-C, free fatty acids, calculated non-HDL-cholesterol and TGs to HDL ratio as well as by a significant increase in HDL-C.

Metformin not only lowers blood glucose concentration but also inhibits adipose tissue lipolysis, reduces circulating levels of FFAs, improves lipid profiles and reduces the rate of formation of advanced glycation end products [167, 311].

The literature showed discrepant results about the influence of metformin on lipid profile [318]. Some studies reported reduction only in TC levels [318, 319], while others reported reduction of TC and TGs with an increase of HDL-C [320, 321]. Still other studies showed no changes in lipid profile [322, 323]. Another investigation showed an association of metformin with an improvement in the lipid profile even in non-diabetic patients [324]. The reasons for these conflicts are not clear, but may be related to the different animal species and models used or different patients' disease profile as well as different dose and duration of metformin treatment.

In accordance to our results, a previous study showed that metformin caused a significant reduction of fasting serum triglycerides, cholesterol and total lipids in STZ diabetic rats [313]. In addition, randomized controlled trials in humans treated with metformin showed a significant reduction in triglycerides and LDL-C as well as an increase in HDL-C [312]. Another study reported that metformin decreased total cholesterol and LDL-C in type 2 diabetic patients intensively treated with insulin. However, non-significant changes in HDL-C and triglycerides were resulted [325]. It was also previously reported that metformin lowered fasting plasma levels of triglycerides, free fatty acids, total cholesterol, LDL and non-HDL cholesterol in patients with type 2 diabetes [326]. In contrast to our work, a previous study showed no effect of metformin on LDL or HDL cholesterol, inspite of the decrease in serum free fatty acids and triglycerides levels in diabetic patients treated with metformin [327].

Furthermore, metformin therapy of type 2 diabetic patients increased LDL particle size and decreased plasma concentrations of remnant lipoprotein cholesterol, which reflects increased atherogenicity. Metformin also decreased the plasma concentrations of methylglyoxal in diabetic patients as well as oxidative stress and related oxidation of LDL[328].

Despite the large number of studies that have established its mode of action, the molecular target of metformin action was elusive for several years until Zhou et al demonstrated in 2001 [329] that metformin treatment activates the energy sensor AMP-activated protein kinase (AMPK), a major cellular regulator of lipid and glucose metabolism, in rat hepatocytes, and thereafter, it was confirmed that metformin treatment stimulates AMPK in tissues in both humans and rodents [314]. AMPK has been identified as a key regulator of cellular energy status [330] and has been implicated in the control of hepatic glucose and lipid homeostasis by many effects on both gene and short term regulation of specific enzymes [331]. It works as an intracellular fuel gauge, which becomes activated in response to a variety of metabolic stresses that typically change the cellular AMP/ATP ratio caused by increasing ATP consumption or reducing ATP production [314]. Thus AMPK activation results in the stimulation of glucose uptake in muscle, fatty acid oxidation in muscle and liver, and the inhibition of hepatic glucose production, cholesterol and triglyceride synthesis, and lipogenesis [330]. Chronic activation of AMPK may also induce the expression of muscle glucose transporter, GLUT4 [329].

Therefore, the increased phosphorylation and activation of AMPK by metformin lead to its beneficial effects on glucose and lipid metabolism. Phosphorylation and inactivation of acetyl-CoA carboxylase (ACC), as a result of AMPK activation, serves to inhibit the rate-limiting step of lipogenesis. Reduced synthesis of the ACC product, malonyl-CoA, is also predicted to increase fatty acid oxidation [329]. Moreover, the synthesis of lipogenic enzymes, along with sterol regulatory element-binding protein 1 (SREBP-1), a key lipogenic transcription factor, is suppressed [149]. These effects are likely to contribute to metformin's in-vivo ability to lower triglycerides and VLDL thus improving dyslipidemia associated with diabetes [329].

The net metformin effect is thus to decrease glucose and lipid synthesis and to increase fat oxidation. The reduced glucose output from the liver and the decrease in ectopic fat accumulation in hepatocytes augment hepatic sensitivity to insulin [332].

The improvement in lipid profile may be not only through the correction of abnormal glucose metabolism in diabetic condition, but also due to an intrinsic potential of metformin to improve lipid abnormalities. Metformin also was reported to cause inhibition of lipid peroxidation and lipoproteins oxidation as well as improvement in antioxidants level in hyperlipidemic rats. All accumulatively indicate a protective effect of metformin against oxidative stress mediated complications [333]. Perhaps this protective effect of metformin may be the cause of the amelioration of lipid profile and oxidative stress parameters seen in our results.

Moreover, our study insured the beneficial effect of metformin treatment on the cardiovascular complications of diabetes by a significant reduction in triglycerides to HDL-cholesterol ratio. This was in accordance to another study which showed a significant reduction in this ratio after metformin treatment [334].

The present study showed that treatment of STZ-diabetic rats with metformin in a dose of 300 mg/kg/day for 2 weeks orally was associated with a significant reduction in lipid peroxidation, reflected by the decrease in hepatic malondialdehyde level, as well as, it caused a significant increase in the antioxidant capacity, revealed by the increase in the hepatic reduced glutathione level as compared to the untreated diabetic rats. This may be due to its antioxidant action and protective effects on the liver.

Previous studies showed that metformin exerts antioxidant activity in streptozotocin-induced diabetic rats [335] and decreases erythrocyte susceptibility to oxidative stress in type 2 diabetic patients [336]. Additionally, when metformin therapy was given to high fructose diet-induced type 2 diabetic rats, it lowered the levels of TBARS and lipid hydroperoxides, decreasing lipid peroxidation as well as it significantly enhanced or maintained the activities of antioxidant enzymes (SOD, CAT, GPx, vitamin E and vitamin C) in the liver of the rats [337].

In another study, metformin treatment resulted in a significant increase in hepatic and kidney GSH content and activities of antioxidant enzymes (SOD, CAT, GST) with significant decrease in TBARS levels in liver and kidney when compared to untreated diabetic rats [338]. Additionally, it was reported that metformin increased the expression of the antioxidant, thioredoxin (Trx), which could mediate some of the metformin's effect on ROS reduction [339].

The drug is known to inhibit oxidative phosphorylation. Although the mechanisms by which this effect is achieved are still not fully known, it was suggested that metformin can enter the mitochondria, accumulate within these organelles and inhibit mildly and specifically the enzymatic activity of complex-1 of the mitochondrial respiratory chain. When islet cells are exposed to metformin, a lower amount of ROS of mitochondrial origin is likely to be produced, which restores a sort of vicious circle, leading to reduced oxidative stress [340]. This is considered an AMPK-independent mechanism through which metformin exerts a direct antioxidant effect [331]. Therefore, metformin, through mitochondrial complex-1 inhibition, can prevent the consequences of oxidative stress on apoptosis and can diminish the mitochondria-related toxicity of hyperglycemia [341]. Thus, beyond its glucose-lowering effects, metformin exhibits antioxidant properties that contribute to the vasculoprotective effects [342]. Furthermore, metformin was reported to possess a direct scavenging effect against oxygenated free radicals generated in-vitro and to decrease intracellular production of ROS in aortic endothelial cells through the reduction of both NAD(P)H oxidase and/or the mitochondrial respiratory chain pathways [343].

The increase of NADPH formation by metformin can be used in regeneration of reduced glutathione by GSH reductase [341], thus reducing intracellular ROS by increasing the activity of the antioxidative glutathione system [339]. A previous study showed that metformin increased glucose-6-phosphate dehydrogenase activity and enhanced the pentose phosphate pathway related formation of NADPH [344].

One of the unique findings in the present study is the anti-inflammatory effect of metformin. The results revealed that treatment of STZ-diabetic rats with metformin was associated with significant decreases in the serum levels of the inflammatory markers; CRP, MCP-1 and NO in comparison to the untreated diabetic rats.

It was reported that metformin might prevent microvascular and macrovascular complications of diabetes mellitus by exhibiting vascular anti-inflammatory and anti-atherogenic activities. Metformin improves vascular endothelial functions, inhibits IL-1β-induced release of the proinflammatory cytokines, improves diabetic dyslipidemia and reduces plasminogen activator inhibitor-1, resulting in subsequent improvement of capillary flow [333]. It was also demonstrated that metformin attenuated the proinflammatory responses in human vascular wall cells and macrophages [345].

However, the detailed molecular mechanisms underlying these anti-inflammatory effects are not fully understood. One study suggested that metformin can exert this anti-inflammatory effect through NF-κB inhibition [346]. Another study showed that metformin attenuated the cytokine-induced expression of proinflammatory and adhesion molecule genes by inhibiting the activation of NF-κB via AMPK activation. In addition, this study showed that metformin inhibited the NF-κB–dependent gene expression of various inflammatory and cell adhesion molecules, including VCAM-1, ICAM-1 and MCP-1 [347]. Recently, it was shown that metformin significantly inhibited TNF production in isolated human monocytes, attenuating the inflammatory responses [345].

Moreover, obese subjects treated with metformin displayed a significant reduction in the inflammatory marker, MCP-1, supporting the hypothesis that metformin can improve the low-grade inflammatory state observed in diabetes [348]. In addition, a previous study showed that in overweight type 2 diabetic patients, metformin reduced the concentration of CRP and regulated it specifically [349]. However, another report showed modest CRP reduction after one year treatment with metformin [350].

In contrast to the results reported in patients with type 2 DM, metformin had no effect on CRP and TNF-α concentrations in patients with impaired glucose tolerance [351], suggesting that metformin, likely, reduces levels of inflammatory markers by reducing hyperglycemia, improving insulin sensitivity, and/or promoting weight loss in patients with T2DM [349].

Furthermore, the anti-inflammatory effects of metformin were demonstrated by iNOS inhibition, resulting in a decrease in serum NO level. Metformin could inhibit iNOS through its well-known mechanism, the AMPK activation, which is believed to contribute to its insulin-sensitizing actions in diabetic subjects. However, inhibition of iNOS induction and reduced NO formation represent a novel mechanism by which metformin improves insulin action in muscle [352].

Previous studies demonstrated the beneficial effects of metformin on the endothelium, which appear to be mediated through its effects to improve insulin resistance. Although, it was suggested that metformin ameliorates endothelial function independently of glycemia. Nevertheless, it is not clear whether these effects are due to the release of endothelial NO or improvement in its signaling as metformin was found to increase endothelial NO levels through phosphorylation of eNOS in cultured endothelium cells [167]. However, several studies have suggested that the vasculoprotective effects of metformin are mainly due to improved NO signaling [298, 311].

Thus, the AMPK activation via metformin inhibits iNOS, which results in decrease in the elevated NO associated with acute hyperglycemia. On the other hand, it improves the endothelial dysfunction, associated with chronic hyperglycemia, by increasing endothelial NO, probably via phosphorylation of eNOS. Eventually, it is intriguing to suggest that metformin does not only improve the metabolic defects in diabetes by increasing glucose uptake and decreasing gluconeogenesis, but additionally protects the vasculature by reducing the oxidative stress and inflammation⁽³⁴¹, ³⁴⁶⁾. Therefore, the unique efficacy of metformin in the treatment of hyperglycemia and insulin resistance dependant complications is presumably not only an expression of one mechanism alone but of the diverse and manifold properties of this old, but useful drug [301, 341].

Interestingly, in our present research, L-cysteine treatment of the STZ-diabetic rats, in a dose of 300 mg/kg/day for 2 weeks orally alone, decreased significantly the levels of fasting serum glucose, insulin and HOMA-IR.

In accordance to our work, a previous study demonstrated that L-cysteine supplementation significantly lowered the circulating levels of plasma glucose and glycated hemoglobin and the HOMA index of insulin resistance in ZDF rats, a model of type 2 diabetes [75]. In addition, previous studies reported lower glucose intolerance and insulin level in high fructose fed rats or in hyperinsulinemic subjects following thiol or sulfur amino acids supplementation [140, 141]. Interestingly, dietary cysteine was also shown to improve glucose control and alleviate sucrose-induced insulin resistance [353].

The resulted improvement in glycemic control and insulin resistance associated with cysteine treatment may be due to a decrease in AGEs formation. It is known that insulin resistance and impaired glucose metabolism can result in the accumulation of reactive aldehydes, including methylglyoxal and glyoxal. These aldehydes react with free SH and amino groups of proteins and DNA to form advanced glycation end products (AGEs). Thiols such as cysteine also bind these aldehydes, allowing them to be excreted in bile and urine. This results in a reduction in the development of diabetic complications [115]. It was demonstrated that AGE-RAGE interaction increased intracellular oxidative stress, causing a decrease in glucose uptake in cultured adipocytes. This effect was completely reversed by cysteine supply [136]. In addition, another study showed that methylglyoxal decreased insulin-induced IRS-1 tyrosine phosphorylation and decreased kinase activity of PI3K, impairing insulin signaling in cultured adipocytes. This impairment was prevented by the addition of N-acetyl cysteine to the cell culture [137].

One of our novel findings is the beneficial effect of L-cysteine treatment on lipid profile as compared to the untreated diabetic rats. L-cysteine treatment of the STZ-diabetic rats in a dose of 300 mg/kg/day for 2 weeks orally resulted in significant reductions in the levels of LDL-C, free fatty acids, calculated non-HDL-cholesterol and triglycerides to HDL-C ratio as well as it significantly increased the serum level of HDL-C. However, L-cysteine did not show any significant reductions in the level of serum triglycerides and total cholesterol.

Our results were in accordance to Diniz et al in 2006 [354], who showed that cysteine supplementation prevented the elevation of oxidized LDL induced by high sucrose intake. They also reported that it had beneficial effects on enhancing HDL/triacylglycerol, reducing cholesterol/HDL and normalizing effectively serum triacylglycerol and VLDL. It is evident that these beneficial effects on serum lipids were related to cysteine's antioxidant property, in both liver and serum, as cysteine promotes the maintenance of protein structure, against oxidation by ROS, facilitating the lipoprotein receptors functions and improving the cellular uptake of serum lipids from the blood [354]. Another earlier study showed that HDL-C was increased by cysteine supplementation; suggesting the possibility that a decrease in serum HDL-cholesterol may be related to changes of the plasma thiol level and/or the thiol/disulfide redox status [355]. However, the molecular mechanisms, by which L-cysteine supplementation improved lipid profile are not fully known. These improvements may reflect a tendency towards an overall improvement in general health and tissue metabolic status [356].

In our present study, we also found that elevated malondialdehyde level in the liver of the STZ-diabetic rats was more decreased by L-cysteine supplementation, in a dose of 300 mg/kg/day for 2 weeks orally, than by metformin, indicating better reduction of lipid peroxidation. Moreover, L-cysteine caused a more significant increase in hepatic reduced glutathione than metformin, suggesting more improvements in oxidative stress.

Previously, Blouet et al in 2007 [139] provided the first demonstration that, under sucrose-induced oxidative stress, increasing cysteine intake markedly prevented postprandial deterioration of the redox status, reported as being a key determinant of the detrimental effects of nutrients in the initiation of diabetes and atherosclerosis. Moreover, previous studies have reported a beneficial effect of cysteine supplementation in the prevention of post-exercise oxidative stress in human subjects [353, 357].

It was also showed that the addition of N-acetylcysteine to drinking water supplied to high sucrose-fed Wistar rats, resulted in increased SOD and GSH levels, glutathione peroxidase activity and the GSH/GSSG ratio [354]. Moreover, Oral NAC given to type 2 diabetic patients increased intraerythrocytic GSH levels and the GSH/GSSG ratio [115].

Using cysteine derivatives or cysteine-rich dietary proteins has been shown to increase blood and intracellular glutathione, which may affect the thiol redox status [353]. Moreover, there is evidence, which may support the idea that the effects of cysteine on glucose and lipid homeostasis are mediated by an increase in hepatic GSH output, which in turn positively affects body redox status and early events of the insulin signaling pathway [139]. As it was shown that the cysteine supply determines decisively the intracellular glutathione concentration of lymphocytes and macrophages thus prevents the LDL oxidation and cellular apoptosis mediated by the decrease in the intracellular GSH concentration [355].

A previous study also showed that cysteine supplementation resulted in the enhancement of the endogenous antioxidant capacity, which was revealed by the decrease in thiobarbituric acid reactive substances (TBARS) [358]. Moreover, it enhanced GSH reductase activity thus shifting NADPH, to reduce GSSG [359]. Another study also showed that increasing dietary cysteine content, dose dependently, increased hepatic GSH. This indicates that hepatic GSH delivery and turnover were increased in rats. This study also showed significant correlations between muscle intracellular redox status and insulin signaling, suggesting that the beneficial effects of cysteine-rich diets on glucose homeostasis may be mediated by their ability to maintain the peripheral GSH status [139].

Cysteine not only provides the cells with the rate-limiting ingredient of GSH, but also helps to maintain other antioxidative molecules in their reduced form. Moreover, it was reported that cysteine reacted directly with H_2O_2 producing a concentration-dependent protective effect against H_2O_2-induced oxidative stress in insulinoma cells. Therefore, these effects were proposed to contribute, at least partly, to the mechanisms by which cysteine improves and maintains β-cell viability and function as well as the integrity of nuclear DNA [295].

In addition to L-cysteine's ability to improve glycemic control, lipid profile and oxidative stress, it caused a significant decrease in CRP, MCP-1 and NO levels, when it was given in a dose of 300 mg/kg/day for 2 weeks orally in comparison to the untreated diabetic group. This reflects L-cysteine's anti-inflammatory effect. This finding was in accordance to a recent study, which showed that L-cysteine supplementation lowered significantly blood levels of CRP and MCP-1 in ZDF rats [75].

It was postulated that the inhibitory effect of L-cysteine on the release of proinflammatory cytokines might be mediated partly by inhibiting oxidative stress pathways. Cysteine could have prevented NF-κB activation, which is a primary inducer of the inflammatory pathway, possibly by inhibiting the glucose-mediated production of ROS, thus reducing MCP-1 and CRP levels. This reduction is likely to increase insulin sensitivity and thereby improving glucose metabolism [75]. This can also explain the observed lowering of blood glucose, insulin and HOMA-IR in L-cysteine supplemented diabetic rats, as observed in our results.

The significant reduction in NO concentration by L-cysteine supplementation seen in our study may be due to the inhibition of iNOS activation. It was reported that cysteine supplementation inhibits the proinflammatory cytokines (TNF-α and IL-1β), blocks the activation of NF-κB and increases the anti-inflammatory cytokine IL-10. The induction of IL-1β and activation of NF-κB were shown to precede the induction of iNOS. Thus through this mechanism, cysteine can inhibit iNOS activation leading to decrease in the elevated NO concentration associated with the inflammatory conditions [360]. It was reported that chronic cysteine supplementation in alloxan induced diabetic mice reduced the activation of

NF-κB in the pancreas with the potential of reducing the production of proinflammatory cytokines such as interleukins and iNOS [361].

A previous study showed that cysteine supplementation, for 3 weeks to diabetic rats, reduced the immunostaining of iNOS as well as nitrotyrosine, which indicated the inhibitions of iNOS activation and peroxynitrite-mediated cytotoxicity. They suggested that the improvement of the diabetic rats by cysteine supply is due to the suppression of oxidative stress, which results in the preservation of proteins, such as receptors, enzymes, transport proteins and structural proteins, as well as reduction of cellular damage through lipid peroxidation. This finding provides evidence that antioxidant therapy offers protection against cellular damage in various animal models of diabetes as well as in diabetic patients and also reveals the strong antioxidant effect of L-cysteine [358].

Nevertheless, as a major endogenous antioxidant, cysteine can improve the endothelial function, as it protects endothelial NO, eNOS and signaling pathways from the oxidative effects of ROS, thereby preserving NO bioavailability. A previous study showed that NAC increased eNOS expression and activity in both bovine and human endothelial cells in culture [362]. Moreover, in type 1 diabetic rats, NAC supplied in drinking water for eight weeks normalized endothelium-dependent vasodilatation in the aorta [363].

It should be noted that, in our study, the antioxidant and anti-inflammatory effects of L-cysteine exceeded that of metformin except on nitric oxide. The effect of metformin on nitric oxide was higher. This may be attributed to the ability of metformin to inhibit the activated iNOS via AMPK activation. However, controversy data suggest that L-cysteine has no or mild inhibitory effect on iNOS after its activation.

The results of the present study also showed that the combination between metformin and L-cysteine, each given in a dose of 300 mg/kg/day for 2 weeks orally, was associated with better significant improvements in all studied parameters than either drug alone as compared to the untreated diabetic rats. This was evidenced by significant decreases in the levels of fasting serum glucose, insulin, calculated HOMA-IR, serum triglycerides, total cholesterol, LDL-C,

free fatty acids, calculated non-HDL-cholesterol, and triglycerides to HDL-C ratio, MCP-1, nitric oxide, CRP and hepatic MDA. In addition, there were significant increases in serum HDL-C and hepatic GSH. On the other side, results of combination treatment were similar to metformin treatment in lowering triglycerides and total cholesterol, suggesting that this lowering is due to the effect of metformin alone. However, the combination treatment was significantly better for all other parameters than the metformin group. In comparison to L-cysteine treated group, the combination treatment was far better in all measured parameters.

The improvements in oxidative stress and anti-inflammatory parameters, seen in the combination group, may be due to combing between two drugs; both have antioxidant and anti-inflammatory activities, resulting in a synergistic effect. This gave better results than either drug used alone. The augmented results seen in combination of metformin and L-cysteine, in terms of further improvement in glycemic control, lipid profile, oxidative stress and inflammation could be, in part, explained by the double inhibiting of NF-κB activation. However, research into the molecular mechanism for the augmented hypoglycemic, antioxidant and anti-inflammatory effects of the combination between metformin and L-cysteine is needed to be further investigated and clinical trials on diabetic patients are needed.

In fact, medical science still has many unknown regions to explore. Therefore, further research will be always needed to help in the evaluation and integration of many remedies and search strategies and to offer a framework that helps in guiding clinical decision making for suitable choice of different medication in different situation for world prosperity.

CONCLUSION AND RECOMMENDATIONS

From the results of the present study, it could be concluded that:

- High fat diet/STZ induced experimental diabetes is a reliable mean for creating an animal model, which mimics type 2 diabetes mellitus in humans. This model represents a good example of type 2 diabetes mellitus, simulating the metabolic derangements, oxidative stress and inflammation that occur in humans. This pattern indicates a harmful effect of STZ, which should be taken into consideration in patients under STZ treatment as an antitumor agent. Besides, it gives a convincing clue that dietary imbalance is an essential factor in both initation and development of type 2 diabetes mellitus.

- Environmental factors, especially the visceral obesity, are implicated in the pathogenesis of type 2 diabetes mellitus.

- Type 2 experimental diabetes is associated with chronic hyperglycemia and elevated free fatty acids that resulted in elevated oxidants and lipid peroxides as well as elevated inflammatory markers. Therefore, the amelioration of oxidative stress and inflammation, besides the glycemic and lipid control in diabetic patients must be taken into consideration in the new therapeutic approaches.

- Diabetes mellitus is associated with characteristic lipid profile, referred to as dyslipidemia triad, which is usually an increase in triglycerides and LDL-cholesterol with a concomitant decrease in HDL-cholesterol.

- Metformin is the gold star of the antidiabetic drugs. The results of the present study show that metformin improves insulin sensitivity and lipid profile as well as it exhibits antioxidant and anti-inflammatory effects, besides its glycemic control property.

- L-cysteine is a promising therapeutic agent, which can correct some of the derangements occurring in type 2 diabetes mellitus, especially the oxidative stress and vascular inflammation. The antioxidant and the anti-inflammatory effects of L-cysteine are more evident than that of metformin, in the improvement of oxidative stress markers, as the reduction of hepatic MDA level and the increase of hepatic GSH level, as well as, in the reduction of the inflammatory markers, serum MCP-1 and CRP. Besides, L-cysteine possesses anti-hyperglycemic effects. These findings are novel and need to be explored in the diabetic patients. If it works as well as this research hints, then cysteine supplementation could be used as an adjuvant therapy for better management of diabetes mellitus.

- The combination of metformin and L-cysteine, in the aforementioned doses, was associated with utmost glycemic control as well as improvement of lipid profile, oxidative stress and inflammation. This combination was more effective than either drug alone in decreasing fasting serum glucose, insulin, atherogenic lipoprotein LDL-C, free fatty acids, MCP-1, CRP, NO and hepatic MDA as well as in raising HDL-C and hepatic GSH. This reveals synergistic effect of this drug combination.

After the present study was completed, we recommend that:

- Nutrient management of the type 2 diabetic patients should be applied, especially using the balanced diet and weight reduction, since obesity, especially resulting from high fat diet, leads to increased visceral fat, resulting in insulin resistance and subsequently type 2 diabetes mellitus.

- Metformin is still a mysterious drug, with a lot to explore about its mechanism and effects. It has a very unique effect on diabetic dyslipidemia. It ameliorates the cardiovascular disease risk that is known to be an important secondary complication of diabetes mellitus. It also exerts antioxidant and anti-inflammatory effects that contribute to better management of diabetes.

- The antioxidants should be used, as an add-on therapy to the commonly used oral antidiabetics, is of great beneficial effect for scavenging free radicals, improving antioxidant status and ameliorating the inflammatory condition associated with diabetes. Moreover, as a result of improving the overall body status and health, antioxidants can exert additional improvement in the glycemic control of the diabetic patients.

- In view of synergistic effects of metformin and L-cysteine, further research should be carried out to adjust the optimum doses of both drugs to be used in combination aiming at achieving maximum glycemic control, target lipid profile and amelioration of both oxidative stress and inflammation in diabetic patients.

- Thus, the present study may be considered an addition to the present knowledge about the new mechanism of actions for both metformin and L-cysteine as antioxidants and anti-inflammatory drugs.

- Still a lot to be known about diabetes, its pathophysiology and its management, which represent challenges for researchers to discover.

SUMMARY

Type 2 diabetes mellitus is now a worldwide epidemic disease; affecting at least 150 million people and is projected to increase to 439 million in 2030. Complex genetic predisposition interplays with sedentary life style to induce a state of insulin resistance, which progresses to glucose intolerance, hyperglycemia and overt type 2 diabetes when the pancreatic β-cells are unable to maintain previously high rate of insulin secretion.

Great evidences demonstrate that chronic hyperglycemia and elevated free fatty acids, seen in diabetic patients, underlie oxidative stress and inflammation, which are known to be implicated in the pathogenesis of diabetes mellitus. This state does not emerge from a single dominant route, but through multiple pathways that provide several targets for therapeutic intervention. Hence, a new potential approach, which is the use of antioxidants and anti-inflammatory agents, may signify a useful pharmacologic overture to the management of diabetes. This approach capitalizes on previous data, obtained from both human and animal studies, implicating lipid oversupply, oxidative stress and chronic inflammation as root causes in the development and exacerbation of insulin resistance and diabetes mellitus.

In view of these facts, the present investigation was undertaken to assess the extent of oxidative stress, the antioxidant defense and inflammatory states in high fat diet/STZ induced diabetic rats and the benefits resulting from the combination of the well-established antihyperglycemic drug, metformin and the antioxidant amino acid, L-cysteine. This study was also designed to reveal the effects of metformin and/or L-cysteine on the glycemic control and lipid profile as well as their ability to improve the oxidative stress and inflammation seen in the high fat diet /STZ model of type 2 diabetes mellitus.

Fifty male albino rats weighing between 170-200 gram were used in the current study. Rats were divided into 5 groups, 10 rats in each. In all groups, except group V, rats were kept on a high fat diet for 2 months, after which rendered diabetic by intravenous injection of 15 mg/kg streptozotocin into the caudal vein. After diabetes was confirmed, drug treatment was carried out for 2 weeks as follows:

Group I: Diabetic rats received distilled water orally and served as untreated diabetic control.

Group II: Diabetic rats treated orally with metformin HCl, in a dose of 300mg/kg/day dissolved in distilled water.

Group III: Diabetic rats treated orally with L-cysteine, in a dose of 300mg/kg/day dissolved in distilled water.

Group IV: Diabetic rats treated orally with both metformin HCl in a dose of 300mg/kg/day and L-cysteine in a dose of 300mg/kg/day.

Group V: Fed conventional rat chow and served as normal non-diabetic control.

After 2 weeks of treatment, 12 hours fasted rats were sacrificed by decapitation. Blood was collected and serum was separated for the determination of the following parameters:
- Fasting glucose level.
- Insulin.
- Triglycerides.
- Total cholesterol.
- HDL-cholesterol.
- LDL-cholesterol.
- Free fatty acids.
- Monocyte chemoattractant protein (MCP-1).
- C-reactive protein (CRP).
- Nitric oxide (NO).
- HOMA-IR, non-HDL-cholesterol and triglycerides to HDL-cholesterol ratio were then calculated using their corresponding equations.

Immediately after collection of blood, livers were excised, washed with ice-cold saline and preserved for the assessment of:
- Malondialdehyde (MDA).
- Reduced glutathione (GSH).
- Protein content.

Results of the present study paralleled the published data on the hyperglycemia, dyslipidemia and the increasingly oxidative stress and inflammatory conditions seen in experimentally induced diabetes.

Our study showed that experimentally induced diabetes mellitus was associated with a statistically significant elevated fasting serum insulin, confirming the presence of insulin resistant state, which was accompanied by a significant elevated fasting serum glucose level. This state mimics the natural progressive history of type 2 diabetes mellitus in humans. The levels of triglycerides, total cholesterol, LDL-cholesterol and free fatty acids as well as the calculated non-HDL-cholesterol and TGs to HDL ratio were also elevated while HDL-cholesterol level was decreased significantly. These findings suggest the deleterious effects of hyperglycemia and insulin resistance in the adipose tissue, seen in the diabetic state.

The results also revealed that type 2 diabetes resulted in a pro-oxidant state manifested by an increase in hepatic MDA, generated by lipid peroxidation, and this is coupled with reduction of GSH, which is a protective thiol antioxidant. Since GSH represents the largest source of cellular reducing equivalents, its decrease could significantly affect the overall cellular redox environment. Moreover, the significantly elevated levels of the inflammatory markers MCP-1, C-reactive protein and nitric oxide indicate that inflammation plays an important key role in the pathogenesis of insulin resistance and diabetes mellitus.

Metformin treated group of rats showed a statistically significant decrease in fasting serum glucose, insulin and significant improvement in insulin resistance. Moreover, it caused significant decreases in triglycerides, total cholesterol, free fatty acids, LDL-C, non- HDL-cholesterol and triglycerides to HDL-C ratio as well as a significant increase in HDL-cholesterol.

This study also demonstrates the antioxidant and the anti-inflammatory effects of metformin, which were suggested by the ability of metformin to decrease hepatic MDA level and to increase hepatic GSH concentration, which reflects its ability to ameliorate the hazardous effects of both lipid peroxidation and oxidative stress states accompanied with diabetes mellitus. As well as its ability to decrease significantly serum MCP-1, CRP and NO, which are known to reflect the overall inflammatory status.

However, L-cysteine treated group of rats showed a more statistically significant protection from oxidative stress and inflammation than metformin. This was in terms of the decrease in hepatic MDA level and the increase in hepatic reduced GSH concentration as well as in the decrease in MCP-1 and CRP. It also showed some improvements in other biochemical parameters include fasting serum glucose, insulin, LDL-C, HDL-C and free fatty acids. However, the effect of metformin on these parameters was more statistically significant than L-cysteine group.

Interestingly, the effects of metformin and L-cysteine combination for 2 weeks on all measured or calculated parameters were more superior as compared to the effects of either drug when used alone, suggesting their synergism. However, the decreases in serum triglycerides and total cholesterol were totally attributable to metformin as L-cysteine showed non-significant effect on both parameters. Taken together, our results indicate that fasting hyperglycemia, hyperinsulinemia, unfavorable lipid profile as well as the oxidative stress and inflammatory states caused by the diabetic state, were improved, in a statistically significant way, to a great extent on giving combination treatment than either drug when used alone.

Thus our results, obtained from the combination of metformin and L-cysteine, confirm the beneficial and protective effects that can be resulted from the use of an antioxidant drug, with anti-inflammatory effect, as an add-on therapy to the well-known antidiabetic drugs used for management and treatment of type 2 diabetes mellitus.

This study is considered as a new addition to the current knowledge about the derangements occurring in type 2 diabetes mellitus and its evaluation. This study also reveals a new mechanism of action for metformin as an anti-inflammatory drug, in addition to its well-known antihyperglycemic effect and its ability to improve dyslipidemia and oxidative stress in type 2 diabetes mellitus.

The study shows that the antioxidant L-cysteine also has anti-inflammatory and antihyperglycemic effects as well as an ability to improve some of the disturbances of the lipid profile present in type 2 diabetes mellitus. This is novel action and needs to be explored in type 1 and type 2 diabetic patients, as it can be used as an adjuvant therapy for the reduction of oxidative stress, vascular inflammation and cardiovascular diseases in diabetic patients.

REFERENCES

1. Pasupathi P, Chandrasekar V, Kumar US. Evaluation of oxidative stress, enzymatic and non-enzymatic antioxidants and metabolic thyroid hormone status in patients with diabetes mellitus. Diabetes Metab Syndr: Clin Res Rev. 2009;3(3):160-5.

2. Kuzuya T, Nakagawa S, Satoh J, Kanazawa Y, Iwamoto Y, Kobayashi M, et al. Report of the Committee on the classification and diagnostic criteria of diabetes mellitus. Diabetes Res Clin Pract. 2002;55(1):65-85.

3. Nader MM, Eissa LA, Gamil NM, Ammar EM. Effect of nitric oxide, vitamin E and selenium on streptozotocin induced diabetic rats. Saudi Pharma J. 2007;15(1):23-32.

4. Tiwari AK, Rao JM. Diabetes mellitus and multiple therapeutic approaches of phytochemicals: Present status and future prospects. Curr Sci. 2002;83(1):30-7.

5. Maraschin JF, Murussi N, Witter V, Silveiro SP. Diabetes mellitus classification. Arq Bras Cardiol. 2010;95(2):e40-7.

6. Herman WH, Aubert RE, Ali MA, Sous ES, Badran A. Diabetes mellitus in Egypt: risk factors, prevalence and future burden. East Mediterr Health J. 1997;3(1):144–8.

7. American Diabetes Association. Diagnosis and Classification of Diabetes Mellitus. Diabetes care. 2011;34 (1):S62-9.

8. Singh SK, Rastogi A. Gestational diabetes mellitus. Diabetes Metab Syndr: Clin Res Rev. 2008;2(3):227-34.

9. Langer O, Yogev Y, Most O, Xenakis EMJ. Gestational diabetes: the consequences of not treating. Am J Obstet Gynecol. 2005;192(4):989-97.

10. Dode MA, dos Santos IS. Non classical risk factors for gestational diabetes mellitus: a systematic review of the literature. Cad Saude Publica. 2009;25(3):S341-59.

11. Jaïdane H, Hober D. Role of coxsackievirus B4 in the pathogenesis of type 1 diabetes. Diabetes Metab. 2008;34(6):537-48.

12. Raha O, Chowdhury S, Dasgupta S, Raychaudhuri P, Sarkar BN, Raju PV, et al. Approaches in type 1 diabetes research: A status report. Int J Diabetes Dev Ctries. 2009;29(2):85-101.

13. Leu JP, Zonszein J. Diagnostic Criteria and Classification of Diabetes, Ch. 7. In: Poretsky L, editor. Principles of Diabetes Mellitus. 2nd ed. New York: Springer; 2009. p. 107-16.

14. Lin Y, Sun Z. Current views on type 2 diabetes. J Endocrinol. 2010;204(1):1-11.

15. El-Mesallamy HO, Kassem DH, El-Demerdash E, Amin AI. Vaspin and visfatin/Nampt are interesting interrelated adipokines playing a role in the pathogenesis of type 2 diabetes mellitus. Metabolism. 2011;60(1):63-70.

16. Rizvi AA. Type 2 diabetes: epidemiologic trends, evolving pathogenic concepts, and recent changes in therapeutic approach. South Med J. 2004;97(11):1079-87.

17. Reddy MA, Natarajan R. Epigenetic mechanisms in diabetic vascular complications. Cardiovasc Res. 2011;90(3):421-9.

18. Liguori A, Puglianiello A, Germani D, Deodati A, Peschiaroli E, Cianfarani S. Epigenetic Changes Predisposing to Type 2 Diabetes in Intrauterine Growth Retardation. Front Endocrin. 2010;1:1-7.

19. Goldberg AD, Allis CD, Bernstein E. Epigenetics: a landscape takes shape. Cell. 2007;128(4):635-8.

20. Jain S, Saraf S. Type 2 diabetes mellitus--Its global prevalence and therapeutic strategies. Diabetes Metab Syndr: Clin Res Rev. 2010;4(1):48-56.

21. Arslanian S. Type 2 diabetes in children: clinical aspects and risk factors. Horm Res. 2000;57(1):19-28.

22. American Diabetes Association. Type 2 diabetes in children and adolescents. Diabetes Care. 2000;23(3):381-9.

23. Alberti G, Zimmet P, Shaw J, Bloomgarden Z, Kaufman F, Silink M. Type 2 diabetes in the young: the evolving epidemic: the international diabetes federation consensus workshop. Diabetes Care. 2004;27(7):1798-811.

24. Young TK, Martens PJ, Taback SP, Sellers EAC, Dean HJ, Cheang M, et al. Type 2 diabetes mellitus in children: prenatal and early infancy risk factors among native Canadians. Arch Pediatr Adolesc Med 2002;156(7):651-5.
25. Tappy L. Adiposity in children born small for gestational age. Int J Obes (Lond). 2006;30(4):S36-40.
26. Breckenridge SM, Cooperberg BA, Arbelaez AM, Patterson BW, Cryer PE. Glucagon, in concert with insulin, supports the postabsorptive plasma glucose concentration in humans. Diabetes. 2007;56(10):2442-8.
27. DeFronzo RA. Pathogenesis of type 2 diabetes mellitus. Med Clin North Am. 2004;88(4):787-835.
28. Bajaj M, DeFronzo RA. Metabolic and molecular basis of insulin resistance. J Nucl Cardiol. 2003;10(3):311-23.
29. Meier JJ. The contribution of incretin hormones to the pathogenesis of type 2 diabetes. Best Pract Res Clin Endocrinol Metab. 2009;23(4):433-41.
30. Andrade-Cetto A, Vázquez RC. Gluconeogenesis inhibition and phytochemical composition of two Cecropia species. J Ethnopharmacol. 2010;130(1):93-7.
31. Eriksson JW. Metabolic stress in insulin's target cells leads to ROS accumulation-a hypothetical common pathway causing insulin resistance. FEBS lett. 2007;581(19):3734-42.
32. Zeyda M, Stulnig TM. Obesity, inflammation, and insulin resistance– a mini-review. Gerontology. 2009;55(4):379-86.
33. Kirk EP, Klein S. Pathogenesis and pathophysiology of the cardiometabolic syndrome. J Clin Hypertens (Greenwich). 2009;11(12):761-5.
34. Kashyap SR, Belfort R, Berria R, Suraamornkul S, Pratipranawatr T, Finlayson J, et al. Discordant effects of a chronic physiological increase in plasma FFA on insulin signaling in healthy subjects with or without a family history of type 2 diabetes. Am J Physiol Endocrinol Metab. 2004;287(3):E537-46.

35. Tripathy D, Mohanty P, Dhindsa S, Syed T, Ghanim H, Aljada A, et al. Elevation of free fatty acids induces inflammation and impairs vascular reactivity in healthy subjects. Diabetes. 2003;52(12):2882-7.

36. Paz K, Hemi R, LeRoith D, Karasik A, Elhanany E, Kanety H, et al. A molecular basis for insulin resistance. Elevated serine/threonine phosphorylation of IRS-1 and IRS-2 inhibits their binding to the juxtamembrane region of the insulin receptor and impairs their ability to undergo insulin-induced tyrosine phosphorylation. J Biol Chem. 1997;272(47):29911-8.

37. Kim JA, Montagnani M, Koh KK, Quon MJ. Reciprocal relationships between insulin resistance and endothelial dysfunction: molecular and pathophysiological mechanisms. Circulation. 2006;113(15):1888-904.

38. Emoto M, Nishizawa Y, Maekawa K, Hiura Y, Kanda H, Kawagishi T, et al. Homeostasis model assessment as a clinical index of insulin resistance in type 2 diabetic patients treated with sulfonylureas. Diabetes care. 1999;22(5):818-22.

39. Abdin AA, Baalash AA, Hamooda HE. Effects of rosiglitazone and aspirin on experimental model of induced type 2 diabetes in rats: focus on insulin resistance and inflammatory markers. J Diabetes Complications. 2010;24(3):168-78.

40. Buchanan TA. Pancreatic beta-cell loss and preservation in type 2 diabetes. Clin Ther. 2003;25(2):B32-46.

41. Wajchenberg BL. β-cell failure in diabetes and preservation by clinical treatment. Endocr Rev. 2007;28(2):187-218.

42. Bays H, Mandarino L, DeFronzo RA. Role of the adipocyte, free fatty acids, and ectopic fat in pathogenesis of type 2 diabetes mellitus: peroxisomal proliferator-activated receptor agonists provide a rational therapeutic approach. J Clin Endocrinol Metab. 2004;89(2):463-78.

43. Stumvoll M, Goldstein BJ, Van Haeften TW. Type 2 diabetes: principles of pathogenesis and therapy. Lancet. 2005;365(9467):1333-46.

44. Dimitriadis G, Boutati E, Raptis SA. The Lipotoxicity and Glucotoxicity Hypothesis in the Metabolic Syndrome and Type 2

Diabetes, Ch.16. In: Ríos MS, Caro FJ, Carraro R, Fuentes JA, editors. The Metabolic Syndrome at the Beginning of the XXI Century A Genetic and Molecular Approach 1st ed. Spain: Elsevier; 2005. p. 271-82.

45. Henry RR. Preventing cardiovascular complications of type 2 diabetes: focus on lipid management. Clinical Diabetes. 2001;19(3):113-20.

46. Carmena R. Type 2 diabetes, dyslipidemia, and vascular risk: rationale and evidence for correcting the lipid imbalance. Am Heart J. 2005;150(5):859-70.

47. Cnop M. Fatty acids and glucolipotoxicity in the pathogenesis of Type 2 diabetes. Biochem Soc Trans. 2008;36(Pt 3):348-52.

48. Bittner V. Non-HDL cholesterol: meaurment, interpretation, and significance. Adv Stud Med. 2007;7(1):8-11.

49. Da Luz PL, Favarato D, Junior JRFN, Lemos P, ChagasI ACP. High ratio of triglycerides to HDL-cholesterol predicts extensive coronary disease. Clinics (Sao Paulo). 2008;64(4):427-32.

50. McLaughlin T, Reaven G, Abbasi F, Lamendola C, Saad M, Waters D, et al. Is there a simple way to identify insulin-resistant individuals at increased risk of cardiovascular disease? Am J Cardiol. 2005;96(3):399-404.

51. Mooradian AD. Dyslipidemia in type 2 diabetes mellitus. Nat Clin Pract Endocrinol Metab. 2009;5(3):150-9.

52. Burant CF. Special therapeutic situations. Medical Management of Type 2 Diabetes. 6th ed. Alexandria: VA: American Diabetes Association, Inc; 2008. p. 87-103.

53. Edmonds ME. Diabetes and its complications, Ch.3. In: Salisburg J, editor. Molecular pathology. 1st ed. USA: Taylor and Francis Inc; 2002. p. 45-73.

54. King KD, Jones JD, Warthen J. Microvascular and macrovascular complications of diabetes mellitus. Am J Pharm Educ. 2005;69(5):1-10.

55. Young BA. Pharmacologic treatment of diabetic nephropathy. Nor Am Pharmacother. 2004;2:50-5.

56. Fong DS, Aiello L, Gardner TW, King GL, Blankenship G, Cavallerano JD, et al. Retinopathy in diabetes. Diabetes Care. 2004;27(1):s84-7.

57. Giacco F, Brownlee M. Oxidative stress and diabetic complications. Circ Res. 2010;107(9):1058-70.

58. Brownlee M. Biochemistry and molecular cell biology of diabetic complications. Nature. 2001;414(6865):813-20.

59. Wautier JL, Schmidt AM. Protein glycation: a firm link to endothelial cell dysfunction. Circ Res. 2004;95(3):233-8.

60. Goldin A, Beckman JA, Schmidt AM, Creager MA. Advanced glycation end products: sparking the development of diabetic vascular injury. Circulation. 2006;114(6):597-605.

61. Veldman BA, Vervoort G. Pathogenesis of renal microvascular complications in diabetes mellitus. Neth J Med. 2002;60(10):390-6.

62. Giacco F, Brownlee M. Pathogenesis of Microvascular Complications, Ch.35. In: Holt RI, Cockram CS, Flyvbjerg A, Goldstein BJ, editors. Textbook of Diabetes. 4th ed: Wiley Blackwell Ltd; 2010. p. 553-74.

63. Kasuga M. Insulin resistance and pancreatic beta cell failure. J Clin Invest. 2006;116(7):1756-60.

64. Anderson JW, Kendall CW, Jenkins DJ. Importance of weight management in type 2 diabetes: review with meta-analysis of clinical studies. J Am Call Nutr. 2003;22(5):331-9.

65. Becker KG. The common variants/multiple disease hypothesis of common complex genetic disorders. Med Hypotheses. 2004;62(2):309-17.

66. Abel ED. Free fatty acid oxidation in insulin resistance and obesity. Heart Metab. 2010;48:5-10.

67. Hajer GR, Van Haeften TW, Visseren FL. Adipose tissue dysfunction in obesity, diabetes, and vascular diseases. Eur Heart J. 2008;29(24):2959-71.

68. Chang YC, Chuang LM. The role of oxidative stress in the pathogenesis of type 2 diabetes: from molecular mechanism to clinical implication. Am J Transl Res. 2010;2(3):316-31.

69. Shoelson SE, Lee J, Goldfine AB. Inflammation and insulin resistance. J Clin Invest. 2006;116(7):1793-801.

70. Singh N, Kafle D, Singh S, Singh AK, Agrawal N. Reactive oxygen species and the role of inflammatory markers (IL-6 and TNF-α) in the causation of insulin resistance in type 2 obese diabetics. Int J Clin Cases Invest. 2010;1(1):1-6.

71. Laaksonen DE, Niskanen L, Nyyssönen K, Punnonen K, Tuomainen TP, Valkonen VP, et al. C-reactive protein and the development of the metabolic syndrome and diabetes in middle-aged men. Diabetologia. 2004;47(8):1403-10.

72. Han KH, Hong KH, Park JH, Ko J, Kang DH, Choi KJ, et al. C-reactive protein promotes monocyte chemoattractant protein-1—mediated chemotaxis through upregulating CC chemokine receptor 2 expression in human monocytes. Circulation. 2004;109(21):2566-71.

73. Jain SK, Rains J, Croad J, Larson B, Jones K. Curcumin supplementation lowers TNF-alpha, IL-6, IL-8, and MCP-1 secretion in high glucose-treated cultured monocytes and blood levels of TNF-alpha, IL-6, MCP-1, glucose, and glycosylated hemoglobin in diabetic rats. Antioxid Redox Signal. 2009;11(2):241-9.

74. Kamei N, Tobe K, Suzuki R, Ohsugi M, Watanabe T, Kubota N, et al. Overexpression of monocyte chemoattractant protein-1 in adipose tissues causes macrophage recruitment and insulin resistance. J Biol Chem. 2006;281(36):26602-14.

75. Jain SK, Velusamy T, Croad JL, Rains JL, Bull R. L-cysteine supplementation lowers blood glucose, glycated hemoglobin, CRP, MCP-1, and oxidative stress and inhibits NF-κB activation in the

livers of Zucker diabetic rats. Free Radic Biol Med. 2009;46(12):1633-8.

76. Pepys MB, Hirschfield GM. C-reactive protein: a critical update. J Clin Invest. 2003;111(12):1805-12.

77. Davì G, Tuttolomondo A, Santilli F, Basili S, Ferrante E, Di Raimondo D, et al. CD40 ligand and MCP-1 as predictors of cardiovascular events in diabetic patients with stroke. J Atheroscler Thromb. 2009;16(6):707-13.

78. Soskić SS, Dobutović BD, Sudar EM, Obradović MM, Nikolić DM, Djordjevic JD, et al. Regulation of inducible nitric oxide synthase (iNOS) and its potential role in insulin resistance, diabetes and heart failure. Open Cardiovasc Med J. 2011;5:153-63.

79. Moussa SA. Oxidative Stress In Diabetes Mellitus. Romanian J Biophys. 2008;18(3):225–36.

80. Ahmed RG. The physiological and biochemical effects of diabetes on the balance between oxidative stress and antioxidant defense system. Med J Islamic World Acad Sci. 2005;15(1):31-42.

81. Karasu Ç. Glycoxidative Stress and Cardiovascular Complications in Experimentally-Induced Diabetes: Effects of Antioxidant Treatment. Open Cardiovasc Med J. 2010;4:240-56.

82. Mohora M, Greabu M, Muscurel C, Du C, Totan A. The sources and the targets of oxidative stress in the etiology of diabetic complications. Romanian J Biophys. 2007;17(2):63-84.

83. Johansen JS, Harris AK, Rychly DJ, Ergul A. Oxidative stress and the use of antioxidants in diabetes: linking basic science to clinical practice. Cardiovasc Diabetol. 2005;4(1):5.

84. Rösen P, Nawroth PP, King G, Möller W, Tritschler HJ, Packer L. The role of oxidative stress in the onset and progression of diabetes and its complications: a summary of a Congress Series sponsored by UNESCO MCBN, the American Diabetes Association and the German Diabetes Society. Diabetes Metab Res Rev. 2001;17(3):189-212.

85. Klaunig JE, Kamendulis LM, Hocevar BA. Oxidative stress and oxidative damage in carcinogenesis. Toxicol Pathol. 2010;38(1):96-109.

86. Valko M, Izakovic M, Mazur M, Rhodes CJ, Telser J. Role of oxygen radicals in DNA damage and cancer incidence. Mol Cell Biochem. 2004;266(1-2):37-56.

87. Pandey KB, Rizvi SI. Markers of oxidative stress in erythrocytes and plasma during aging in humans. Oxid Med Cell Longev. 2010;3(1):2-12.

88. Cheeseman KH, Slater TF. An introduction to free radical biochemistry. Br Med Bull. 1993;49(3):481-93.

89. Valko M, Leibfritz D, Moncol J, Cronin MT, Mazur M, Telser J. Free radicals and antioxidants in normal physiological functions and human disease. Int J Biochem Cell Biol. 2007;39(1):44-84.

90. Sen S, Chakraborty R, Sridhar C, Reddy YS, De B. Free radicals, antioxidants, diseases and phytomedicines: Current status and future prospect. Int J Pharm Sci Rev Res. 2010;3(1):91-100.

91. Halliwell B, Chirico S. Lipid peroxidation: its mechanism, measurement, and significance. Am J Clin Nutr. 1993;57(5):715S-25S.

92. Slatter DA, Bolton CH, Bailey AJ. The importance of lipid-derived malondialdehyde in diabetes mellitus. Diabetologia. 2000;43(5):550-7.

93. Santamaría A, Sánchez-Rodríguez J, Zugasti A, Martínez A, Galván-Arzate S, Segura-Puertas L. A venom extract from the sea anemone Bartholomea annulata produces haemolysis and lipid peroxidation in mouse erythrocytes. Toxicology. 2002;173(3):221-8.

94. Salem M, Kholoussi S, Kholoussi N, Fawzy R. Malondialdehyde and trace element levels in patients with type 2 diabetes mellitus. Arch Hell Med. 2011;28(1):83-8.

95. Onyango AN, Baba N. New hypotheses on the pathways of formation of malondialdehyde and isofurans. Free Radic Biol Med. 2010;49(10):1594-600.

96. Adly AA. Oxidative stress and disease: an update review. Res J Immunol. 2010;3(2):129-45.

97. Wiernsperger NF. Oxidative stress as a therapeutic target in diabetes: revisiting the controversy. Diabetes Metab. 2003;29(6):579-85.

98. Mehta JL, Rasouli N, Sinha AK, Molavi B. Oxidative stress in diabetes: a mechanistic overview of its effects on atherogenesis and myocardial dysfunction. Int J Biochem Cell Biol. 2006;38(5-6):794-803.

99. Puddu P, Puddu GM, Cravero E, De Pascalis S, Muscari A. The emerging role of cardiovascular risk factor-induced mitochondrial dysfunction in atherogenesis. J Biomed Sci. 2009;16(1):1-9.

100. Maritim AC, Sanders RA, Watkins III JB. Diabetes, oxidative stress, and antioxidants: a review. J Biochem Mol Toxicol. 2003;17(1):24-38.

101. Pavlatou MG, Papastamataki M, Apostolakou F, Papassotiriou I, Tentolouris N. FORT and FORD: two simple and rapid assays in the evaluation of oxidative stress in patients with type 2 diabetes mellitus. Metabolism. 2009;58(11):1657-62.

102. Rains JL, Jain SK. Oxidative stress, insulin signaling and diabetes. Free Radic Biol Med. 2011;50(5):567-75.

103. Kirkinezos IG, Moraes CT. Reactive oxygen species and mitochondrial diseases. Semin Cell Dev Biol. 2001;12(6):449-57.

104. Timimi FK, Ting HH, Haley EA, Roddy MA, Ganz P, Creager MA. Vitamin C improves endothelium-dependent vasodilation in patients with insulin-dependent diabetes mellitus. J Am Coll Cardiol. 1998;31(3):552-7.

105. May JM, Qu Z, Neel DR, Li X. Recycling of vitamin C from its oxidized forms by human endothelial cells. Biochim Biophys Acta. 2003;1640(2-3):153-61.

106. Amatyakul S, Chakraphan D, Chotpaibulpan S, Patumraj S. The effect of long-term supplementation of vitamin C on pulpal blood flow in streptozotocin-induced diabetic rats. Clin Hemorheol Microcirc. 2003;29(3-4):313-9.

107. Bleys J, Navas-Acien A, Guallar E. Serum selenium and diabetes in US adults. Diabetes Care. 2007;30(4):829-34.

108. Beckett GJ, Arthur JR. Selenium and endocrine systems. J Endocrinol. 2005;184(3):455-65.

109. Kornhauser C, Garcia-Ramirez JR, Wrobel K, Pérez-Luque EL, Garay-Sevilla M, Wrobel K. Serum selenium and glutathione peroxidase concentrations in type 2 diabetes mellitus patients. Prim Care Diabetes. 2008;2(2):81-5.

110. Wiernsperger N, Rapin JR. Trace elements in glucometabolic disorders: an update. Diabetol Metab Syndr. 2010;2(1):1-9.

111. Morris BW, Blumsohn A, Mac Neil S, Gray TA. The trace element chromium--a role in glucose homeostasis. Am J Clin Nutr. 1992;55(5):989-91.

112. Srivastava AK, Mehdi MZ. Insulino-mimetic and anti-diabetic effects of vanadium compounds. Diabet Med. 2005;22(1):2-13.

113. Khan H, Khan MF, Jan SU, Khan KA, Shah SU. Study of the chemical and metabolic changes in plasma glutathione (GSH) of human blood after lithium introduction. J App Pharm. 2011;2(3):201-11.

114. Perricone C, De Carolis C, Perricone R. Glutathione: a key player in autoimmunity. Autoimmun Rev. 2009;8(8):697-701.

115. Vasdev S, Singal P, Gill V. The antihypertensive effect of cysteine. Int J Angiol. 2009;18(1):7-21.

116. Pastore A, Federici G, Bertini E, Piemonte F. Analysis of glutathione: implication in redox and detoxification. Clin Chim Acta. 2003;333(1):19-39.

117. Kidd PM. Glutathione: systemic protectant against oxidative and free radical damage. Altern Med Rev. 1997;2(3):155-76.

118. Liu S, Sun HX, Briegel JR, Murray A, Sun ZH, Tan ZL, et al. The interaction of blood glutathione concentration and selenium supplementation on the redox states in skeletal muscles, whole body cysteine metabolism and lipid peroxidation in Merino lambs. Trends Anim Vet Sci J. 2010;1(2):65-74.

119. Lu SC. Regulation of glutathione synthesis. Mol Aspects Med. 2009;30(1-2):42-59.
120. Holmgren A, Sengupta R. The use of thiols by ribonucleotide reductase. Free Radic Biol Med. 2010;49(11):1617-28.
121. Kovačević TB, Borković SS, Z. PS, Despotović SG, Saičić ZS. Glutathione as a suitable biomarker in hepatopancreas, gills and muscle of three freshwater crayfish species. Arch Biol Sci. 2008;60(1):59-66.
122. Chakravarthi S, Jessop CE, Bulleid NJ. The role of glutathione in disulphide bond formation and endoplasmic-reticulum-generated oxidative stress. EMBO Rep. 2006;7(3):271-5.
123. Ortega AL, Mena S, Estrela JM. Glutathione in cancer cell death. Cancers. 2011;3(1):1285-310.
124. Anon. Glutathione, reduced (GSH). Monograph. Altern Med Rev. 2001;6(6):601-7.
125. Cacciatore I, Cornacchia C, Pinnen F, Mollica A, Di Stefano A. Prodrug approach for increasing cellular glutathione levels. Molecules. 2010;15(3):1242-64.
126. Dröge W. Oxidative stress and ageing: is ageing a cysteine deficiency syndrome? Philos Trans R Soc Lond B Biol Sci. 2005;360(1464):2355-72.
127. Dominy JE, Stipanuk MH. New roles for cysteine and transsulfuration enzymes: production of H2S, a neuromodulator and smooth muscle relaxant. Nutr Rev. 2004;62(9):348-53.
128. Biçer E, Çetinkaya P. A voltammetric study on the interacton of novobiocin with cysteine: pH effect. J Chil Chem Soc. 2009;54(1):46-50.
129. Kitabatake M, So MW, Tumbula DL, Söll D. Cysteine biosynthesis pathway in the archaeon Methanosarcina barkeri encoded by acquired bacterial genes? J Bacteriol. 2000;182(1):143-5.
130. Tzanavaras PD. Automated determination of pharmaceutically and biologically active thiols by sequential injection analysis: A review. Open Chem Biomed Methods J. 2010;3:37-45.

131. Tang D, Kang R, Zeh III HJ, Lotze MT. High-mobility group box 1, oxidative stress, and disease. Antioxid Redox Signal. 2011;14(7):1315-35.

132. Baker DH, Czarnecki-Maulden GL. Pharmacologic role of cysteine in ameliorating or exacerbating mineral toxicities. J Nutr. 1987;117(6):1003-10.

133. Sprince H, Parker CM, Smith GG, Gonzales LJ. Protection against acetaldehyde toxicity in the rat by L-cysteine, thiamin and L-2-methylthiazolidine-4-carboxylic acid. Agents Actions. 1974;4(2):125-30.

134. Giles NM, Watts AB, Giles GI, Fry FH, Littlechild JA, Jacob C. Metal and redox modulation of cysteine protein function. Chem Biol. 2003;10(8):677-93.

135. Gazit V, Ben-Abraham R, Vofsi O, Katz Y. L-cysteine increases glucose uptake in mouse soleus muscle and SH-SY5Y cells. Metab Brain Dis. 2003;18(3):221-31.

136. Unoki H, Bujo H, Yamagishi S, Takeuchi M, Imaizumi T, Saito Y. Advanced glycation end products attenuate cellular insulin sensitivity by increasing the generation of intracellular reactive oxygen species in adipocytes. Diabetes Res Clin Pract. 2007;76(2):236-44.

137. Jia X, Wu L. Accumulation of endogenous methylglyoxal impaired insulin signaling in adipose tissue of fructose-fed rats. Mol Cell Biochem. 2007;306(1-2):133-9.

138. Ammon HP, Hehl KH, Enz G, Setiadi-Ranti A, Verspohl EJ. Cysteine analogues potentiate glucose-induced insulin release in vitro. Diabetes. 1986;35(12):1390-6.

139. Blouet C, Mariotti F, Azzout-Marniche D, Mathé V, Mikogami T, Tomé D, et al. Dietary cysteine alleviates sucrose-induced oxidative stress and insulin resistance. Free Radic Biol Med. 2007;42(7):1089-97.

140. Song D, Hutchings S, Pang CC. Chronic N-acetylcysteine prevents fructose-induced insulin resistance and hypertension in rats. Eur J Pharmacol. 2005;508(1-3):205-10.

141. Fulghesu AM, Ciampelli M, Muzj G, Belosi C, Selvaggi L, Ayala GF, et al. N-acetyl-cysteine treatment improves insulin sensitivity in women with polycystic ovary syndrome. Fertil Steril. 2002;77(6):1128-35.

142. Horie T, Sakaida I, Yokoya F, Nakajo M, Sonaka I, Okita K. L-cysteine administration prevents liver fibrosis by suppressing hepatic stellate cell proliferation and activation. Biochem Biophys Res Commun. 2003;305(1):94-100.

143. Chen W, Kennedy DO, Kojima A, Matsui-Yuasa I. Polyamines and thiols in the cytoprotective effect of L-cysteine and L-methionine on carbon tetrachloride-induced hepatotoxicity. Amino Acids. 2000;18(4):319-27.

144. Dröge W, Breitkreutz R. Glutathione and immune function. Proc Nutr Soc. 2000;59(4):595-600.

145. Dröge W. Cysteine and glutathione deficiency in AIDS patients: a rationale for the treatment with N-acetyl-cysteine. Pharmacology. 1993;46(2):61-5.

146. Marcucci R, Brunelli T, Giusti B, Fedi S, Pepe G, Poli D, et al. The role of cysteine and homocysteine in venous and arterial thrombotic disease. Am J Clin Pathol. 2001;116(1):56-60.

147. Atkuri KR, Mantovani JJ, Herzenberg LA, Herzenberg LA. N-Acetylcysteine--a safe antidote for cysteine/glutathione deficiency. Curr Opin Pharmacol. 2007;7(4):355-9.

148. Zafarullah M, Li WQ, Sylvester J, Ahmad M. Molecular mechanisms of N-acetylcysteine actions. Cell Mol Life Sci. 2003;60(1):6-20.

149. Evans JL, Youngren JF, Goldfine ID. Effective treatments for insulin resistance: trim the fat and douse the fire. Trends Endocrinol Metab. 2004;15(9):425-31.

150. ICMR-WHO workshop. Non-pharmacological management of diabetes, section 6. Guidelines for Management of Type 2 Diabetes; 2nd-4th May 2003; Chennai2005. p. 11-5.

151. American Diabetes Association, Bantle JP, Wylie-Rosett J, Albright AL, Apovian CM, Clark NG, et al. Nutrition recommendations and

interventions for diabetes: a position statement of the American Diabetes Association. Diabetes care. 2008;31(1):S61-78.

152. Garg M, Garg C. Scientific alternative approach in diabetes-An overview. Phcog Rev. 2008;2(4):284-301.

153. Nyenwe EA, Jerkins TW, Umpierrez GE, Kitabchi AE. Management of type 2 diabetes: evolving strategies for the treatment of patients with type 2 diabetes. Metabolism. 2011;60(1):1-23.

154. Bailey CJ, Krentz AJ. Oral Antidiabetic Agents, Ch.29. In: Holt RI, Cockram CS, Flyvbjerg A, Goldstein BJ, editors. Textbook of diabetes. 4th ed: Wiley Blackwell Ltd; 2010. p. 452-77.

155. Witters LA. The blooming of the French lilac. J Clin Invest. 2001;108(8):1105-7.

156. Bailey CJ, Turner RC. Metformin. N Engl J Med. 1996;334(9):574-9.

157. Hundal RS, Inzucchi SE. Metformin: new understandings, new uses. Drugs. 2003;63(18):1879-94.

158. Stumvoll M, Häring HU, Matthaei S. Metformin. Endocr Res. 2007;32(1-2):39-57.

159. Zangeneh F, Kudva YC, Basu A. Insulin sensitizers. Mayo Clin Proc. 2003;78(4):471-9.

160. Green J, Feinglos M. New combination treatments in the management of diabetes: focus on sitagliptin–metformin. Vasc Health Risk Manag. 2008;4(4):743-51.

161. Lim CT, Kola B, Korbonits M. AMPK as a mediator of hormonal signalling. J Mol Endocrinol. 2010;44(2):87-97.

162. Maida A, Lamont BJ, Cao X, Drucker DJ. Metformin regulates the incretin receptor axis via a pathway dependent on peroxisome proliferator-activated receptor-α in mice. Diabetologia. 2011;54(2):339-49.

163. Cheng JT, Huang CC, Liu IM, Tzeng TF, Chang CJ. Novel mechanism for plasma glucose-lowering action of metformin in streptozotocin-induced diabetic rats. Diabetes. 2006;55(3):819-25.

164. Scarpello JH, Howlett HC. Metformin therapy and clinical uses. Diab Vasc Dis Res. 2008;5(3):157-67.

165. Wiernsperger NF. 50 years later: is metformin a vascular drug with antidiabetic properties? Br J Diabetes Vasc Dis 2007;7(5):204-10.

166. Hsieh CH, He CT, Lee CH, Wu LY, Hung YJ. Both slow-release and regular-form metformin improve glycemic control without altering plasma visfatin level in patients with type 2 diabetes mellitus. Metabolism. 2007;56(8):1087-92.

167. Nathanson D, Nyström T. Hypoglycemic pharmacological treatment of type 2 diabetes: targeting the endothelium. Mol Cell Endocrinol. 2009;297(1-2):112-26.

168. Memişoğullari R, Türkeli M, Bakan E, Akçay F. Effect of metformin or gliclazide on lipid peroxidation and antioxidant levels in patients with diabetes mellitus. Turk J Med Sci. 2008;38(6):545-8.

169. Sheehan MT. Current therapeutic options in type 2 diabetes mellitus: a practical approach. Clin Med Res. 2003;1(3):189-200.

170. Fowler MJ. Diabetes Treatment: Oral Agents. Clin Diabetes. 2010;28(3):132-6.

171. Al Awadhi SS, Clifford RM, Sunderland VB, Hackett LRP, Farah H, Shareef TM. Do contraindications to metformin therapy deprive type 2 diabetic patients of its benefits? Int J Diabetes & Metabolism. 2008;16:81-4.

172. Joshi P, Joshi S. Oral hypoglycaemic drugs and newer agents use in type 2 diabetes mellitus. SA Pharmaceutical J. 2008;75(9):38-43.

173. Stafford JM, Elasy T. Treatment update: thiazolidinediones in combination with metformin for the treatment of type 2 diabetes. Vasc Health Risk Manag. 2007;3(4):503-10.

174. Rizos CV, Liberopoulos EN, Mikhailidis DP, Elisaf MS. Pleiotropic effects of thiazolidinediones. Expert Opin Pharmacother. 2008;9(7):1087-108.

175. Rachek LI, Yuzefovych LV, Ledoux SP, Julie NL, Wilson GL. Troglitazone, but not rosiglitazone, damages mitochondrial DNA and

induces mitochondrial dysfunction and cell death in human hepatocytes. Toxicol Appl Pharmacol. 2009;240(3):348-54.

176. Akiyama TE, Meinke PT, Berger JP. PPAR ligands: potential therapies for metabolic syndrome. Curr Diab Rep. 2005;5(1):45-52.

177. Cohen D. Rosiglitazone: what went wrong? BMJ. 2010;341:530-7.

178. Leyvraz C, Suter M, Verdumo C, Calmes JM, Paroz A, Darimont C, et al. Selective effects of PPAR-γ agonists and antagonists on human pre-adipocyte differentiation. Diabetes Obes Metab. 2010;12(3):195-203.

179. Muhlhausler B, Smith SR. Early-life origins of metabolic dysfunction: role of the adipocyte. Trends Endocrinol Metab. 2009;20(2):51-7.

180. Tack CJ, Smits P. Thiazolidinedione derivatives in type 2 diabetes mellitus. Neth J Med. 2006;64(6):166-74.

181. Cusi K. Nonalcoholic fatty liver disease in type 2 diabetes mellitus. Curr Opin Endocrinol Diabetes Obes. 2009;16(2):141-9.

182. Bailey CJ, Day C. Thiazolidinediones today. Br J Diabetes Vasc Dis. 2001;1(1):7-13.

183. Krentz AJ, Bailey CJ. Oral antidiabetic agents: current role in type 2 diabetes mellitus. Drugs. 2005;65(3):385-411.

184. Rhee MK, Umpierrez GE. Improving Insulin Sensitivity: A Review of New Therapies. Clin Cornerstone. 2008;9(2):S28-38.

185. Bösenberg LH, van Zyl DG. The mechanism of action of oral antidiabetic drugs: A review of recent literature. JEMDSA. 2008;13(3):80-8.

186. Wadkar KA, Magdum CS, Patil SS, Naikwade NS. Anti-diabetic potential and indian medicinal plants. J Herb Med Toxicol. 2008;2(1):45-50.

187. Maloff BL, Lockwood DH. In vitro effects of a sulfonylurea on insulin action in adipocytes. Potentiation of insulin-stimulated hexose transport. J Clin Invest. 1981;68(1):85-90.

188. Kanda Y, Matsuda M, Tawaramoto K, Kawasaki F, Hashiramoto M, Matsuki M, et al. Effects of sulfonylurea drugs on adiponectin production from 3T3-L1 adipocytes: implication of different mechanism from pioglitazone. Diabetes Res Clin Pract. 2008;81(1):13-8.

189. Inzucchi SE. Oral antihyperglycemic therapy for type 2 diabetes: scientific review. JAMA. 2002;287(3):360-72.

190. Tentolouris N, Voulgari C, Katsilambros N. A review of nateglinide in the management of patients with type 2 diabetes. Vasc Health Risk Manag. 2007;3(6):797-807.

191. Dornhorst A. Insulinotropic meglitinide analogues. Lancet. 2001;358(9294):1709-16.

192. Whittaker C. A review of oral diabetic medication. SA Pharmaceutical J. 2010;77(6):20-5.

193. Blicklé JF. Meglitinide analogues: a review of clinical data focused on recent trials. Diabetes Metab. 2006;32(2):113-20.

194. Desai A, Tandon N. Management of type 2 diabetes mellitus with oral antihyperglycaemic therapy. Natl Med J India. 2007;20(4):192-8.

195. Hirose T, Miyashita Y, Takagi M, Sumitani S, Kouhara H, Kasayama S. Characteristics of type 2 diabetic patients responding to voglibose administration as an adjunct to sulfonylurea. Diabetes Res Clin Pract. 2001;54(1):9-15.

196. Harrigan RA, Nathan MS, Beattie P. Oral agents for the treatment of type 2 diabetes mellitus: pharmacology, toxicity, and treatment. Ann Emerg Med. 2001;38(1):68-78.

197. Campbell RK, Cobble ME, Reid TS, Shomali ME. Distinguishing among incretin-based therapies. Pathophysiology of type 2 diabetes mellitus: potential role of incretin-based therapies. J Fam Pract. 2010;59(9 Suppl 1):S5-9.

198. Green B, Flatt P, Bailey C. Gliptins: DPP-4 inhibitors to treat type 2 diabetes. Future Prescriber. 2007;8(3):6-12.

199. White JR. Dipeptidyl peptidase-IV inhibitors: pharmacological profile and clinical use. Clin Diabetes. 2008;26(2):53-7.

200. Gerich J. DPP-4 inhibitors: what may be the clinical differentiators? Diabetes Res Clin Pract. 2010;90(2):131-40.

201. Flatt PR, Bailey CJ, Green BD. Dipeptidyl peptidase IV (DPP IV) and related molecules in type 2 diabetes. Front Biosci. 2008;13:3648-60.

202. Neff LM, Kushner RF. Emerging role of GLP-1 receptor agonists in the treatment of obesity. Diabetes Metab Syndr Obes. 2010;3:263-73.

203. Pratley RE, Gilbert M. Targeting incretins in type 2 diabetes: role of GLP-1 receptor agonists and DPP-4 inhibitors. Rev Diabet Stud. 2008;5(2):73-94.

204. Barnett AH. New treatments in type 2 diabetes: a focus on the incretin based therapies. Clin Endocrinol (Oxf). 2009;70(3):343-53.

205. Madsbad S. Exenatide and liraglutide: different approaches to develop GLP-1 receptor agonists (incretin mimetics)-preclinical and clinical results. Best Pract Res Clin Endocrinol Metab. 2009;23(4):463-77.

206. Gallwitz B. The evolving place of incretin-based therapies in type 2 diabetes. Pediatr Nephrol. 2010;25(7):1207-17.

207. Bush MA, Matthews JE, De Boever EH, Dobbins RL, Hodge RJ, Walker SE, et al. Safety, tolerability, pharmacodynamics and pharmacokinetics of albiglutide, a long acting glucagon like peptide-1 mimetic, in healthy subjects. Diabetes Obes Metab. 2009;11(5):498-505.

208. Baggio LL, Huang Q, Brown TJ, Drucker DJ. A recombinant human glucagon-like peptide (GLP)-1–albumin protein (albugon) mimics peptidergic activation of GLP-1 receptor-dependent pathways coupled with satiety, gastrointestinal motility, and glucose homeostasis. Diabetes. 2004;53(9):2492-500.

209. Nauck MA, Ratner RE, Kapitza C, Berria R, Boldrin M, Balena R. Treatment with the human once-weekly glucagon-like peptide-1 analog taspoglutide in combination with metformin improves glycemic control and lowers body weight in patients with type 2

diabetes inadequately controlled with metformin alone: a double-blind placebo-controlled study. Diabetes Care. 2009;32(7):1237-143.

210. Christensen M, Knop FK, Holst JJ, Vilsbøll T. Lixisenatide, a novel GLP-1 receptor agonist for the treatment of type 2 diabetes mellitus. IDrugs. 2009;12(8):503-13.

211. Edelman S, Maier H, Wilhelm K. Pramlintide in the treatment of diabetes mellitus. BioDrugs. 2008;22(6):375-86.

212. Messer C, Green D. A review of Pramlintide in the management of diabetes. Clin Med Ther. 2009;1:305-11.

213. Ryan GJ, Jobe LJ, Martin R. Pramlintide in the treatment of type 1 and type 2 diabetes mellitus. Clin Ther. 2005;27(10):1500-12.

214. Ryan G, Briscoe TA, Jobe L. Review of pramlintide as adjunctive therapy in treatment of type 1 and type 2 diabetes. Drug Des Devel Ther. 2009;2:203-14.

215. Srinivasan BT, Jarvis J, Khunti K, Davies MJ. Recent advances in the management of type 2 diabetes mellitus: a review. Postgrad Med J. 2008;84(996):524-31.

216. Van Gaal LF, Rissanen AM, Scheen AJ, Ziegler O, Rössner S. Effects of the cannabinoid-1 receptor blocker rimonabant on weight reduction and cardiovascular risk factors in overweight patients: 1-year experience from the RIO-Europe study. Lancet. 2005;365(9468):1389-97.

217. Le Foll B, Gorelick DA, Goldberg SR. The future of endocannabinoid-oriented clinical research after CB1 antagonists. Psychopharmacology (Berl). 2009;205(1):171-4.

218. Seewoodhary J, Thornton J, Bain SC. Experimental agents in type 2 diabetes: The next 20 years. WLMJ. 2010;2(3):29-36.

219. Bastaki S. Diabetes mellitus and its treatment. Int J Diabetes Metab. 2005;13(3):111-34.

220. Binder C, Brange J. Insulin chemistry and pharmacokinetics. In: Porte D, Sherwin RS, editors. Ellenberg's and Rifkin's Diabetes Mellitus. 5th ed. Stamford, CT Appleton and Lange; 1997 p. 689.

221. Fung M, Tildesley HD, Gill S. New treatments and treatment philosophy for type 1 diabetes. BCMJ. 2004;46(9):451-6.

222. Nolte MS, Karam JH. Pancreatic hormones and antidiabetic drugs, Ch.41. In: Katzung BG, editor. Basic and clinical pharmacology. 10th ed. New York: Lange Medical Books/McGraw-Hill; 2007. p. 683-703.

223. Unger J. Physiologic insulin replacement therapy. Diabetes Management in Primary Care. 1st ed. Philadelphia, PA: Lippincott, Williams and Wilkins; 2007. p. 192-264.

224. Mayfield JA, White RD. Insulin therapy for type 2 diabetes: rescue, augmentation, and replacement of beta-cell function. Am Fam Physician. 2004;70(3):489-500.

225. Rang HP, Dale MM, Ritter JM, Flower RJ. The endocrine pancreas and the control of blood glucose. Pharmacology Textbook, Ch 25. 6th ed. Edinburgh: Churchill Livingstone; 2007. p. 397-409.

226. Belfiore F, Iannello S. Insulin treatment in Type 1 andType 2 diabetes: Practical goals and algorithms. In: Belfiore F, Mogensen CE, editors. New Concept in Diabetes and its Treatment. Switzerland: Karger AG, Basel; 2000 p. 72-89.

227. Meetoo D, Lappin M. Nanotechnology and the future of diabetes management. J Diabetes Nurs. 2009;13(8):288-97.

228. Sajeesh S, Sharma CP. Cyclodextrin-insulin complex encapsulated polymethacrylic acid based nanoparticles for oral insulin delivery. Int J Pharm. 2006;325(1-2):147-54.

229. Mooradian AD, Bernbaum M, Albert SG. Narrative review: a rational approach to starting insulin therapy. Ann Intern Med. 2006;145(2):125-34.

230. Wada T, Azegami M, Sugiyama M, Tsuneki H, Sasaoka T. Characteristics of signalling properties mediated by long-acting insulin analogue glargine and detemir in target cells of insulin. Diabetes Res Clin Pract. 2008;81(3):269-77.

231. Demssie YN, Younis N, Soran H. The role of insulin detemir in overweight type 2 diabetes management. Vasc Health Risk Manag. 2009;5(3):553-60.

232. Zinman B, Fulcher G, Rao PV, Thomas N, Endahl LA, Johansen T, et al. Insulin degludec, an ultra-long-acting basal insulin, once a day or three times a week versus insulin glargine once a day in patients with type 2 diabetes: a 16-week, randomised, open-label, phase 2 trial. Lancet. 2011;377(9769):924-31.

233. Cheng AY, Zinman B. Principles of insulin therapy, Ch. 39. In: Kahn CR, Weir GC, King GL, editors. Joslin's Diabetes Mellitus. Boston, MA: Lippincott Williams & Wilkins; 2005. p. 559–670.

234. Isaev NK, Stel'mashuk EV, Zorov DB. Cellular mechanisms of brain hypoglycemia. Biochemistry (Mosc). 2007;72(5):471-8.

235. Radermecker RP, Piérard GE, Scheen AJ. Lipodystrophy reactions to insulin: effects of continuous insulin infusion and new insulin analogs. Am J Clin Dermatol. 2007;8(1):21-8.

236. Burant CF. Detection and treatment of chronic complications. Medical Management of Type 2 Diabetes. 6th ed. Alexandria: VA: American Diabetes Association, Inc; 2008. p. 105-37.

237. Zhang F, Ye C, Li G, Ding W, Zhou W, Zhu H, et al. The rat model of type 2 diabetic mellitus and its glycometabolism characters. Exp Anim. 2003;52(5):401-7.

238. Sartoretto JL, Melo GA, Carvalho MH, Nigro D, Passaglia RT, Scavone C, et al. Metformin treatment restores the altered microvascular reactivity in neonatal streptozotocin-induced diabetic rats increasing NOS activity, but not NOS expression. Life Sci. 2005;77(21):2676-89.

239. Liu Z, Li J, Zeng Z, Liu M, Wang M. The antidiabetic effects of cysteinyl metformin, a newly synthesized agent, in alloxan-and streptozocin-induced diabetic rats. Chem Biol Interact. 2008;173(1):68-75.

240. Barham D, Trinder P. An improved colour reagent for the determination of blood glucose by the oxidase system. Analyst. 1972;97(1151):142-5.

241. Bank HL. A quantitative enzyme-linked immunosorbent assay for rat insulin. J Immunoassay. 1988;9(2):135-58.

242. Rifai N, Bachorik PS, Albers JJ. Lipids, lipoproteins and apolipoproteins. In: Burtis CA, Ashwood ER, WB, editors. Tietz Textbook of Clinical Chemistry. 3rd ed. Philadelphia Sauders Co; 1999. p. 809-61.

243. Allain CC, Poon LS, Chan CSG, Richmond W, Fu PC. Enzymatic determination of total serum cholesterol. Clin Chem. 1974;20(4):470-5.

244. Grove TH. Effect of reagent pH on determination of high-density lipoprotein cholesterol by precipitation with sodium phosphotungstate-magnesium. Clin Chem. 1979;25(4):560-4.

245. Friedewald WT, Levy RI, Fredrickson DS. Estimation of the concentration of low-density lipoprotein cholesterol in plasma, without use of the preparative ultracentrifuge. Clinical Chemistry. 1972;18(6):499-502.

246. Shimizu S, Tani Y, Yamada H, Tabata M, Murachi T. Enzymatic determination of serum-free fatty acids: a colorimetric method. Anal Biochem. 1980;107(1):193-8.

247. Evanoff HL, Burdick MD, Moore SA, Kunkel SL, Strieter RM. A sensitive ELISA for the detection of monocyte chemoattractant protein-1 (MCP-1). Immunol Invest. 1992;21(1):39-45.

248. Chan DW, Perlstein MT. Immunoassay: A practical guide. New York: Academic Press; 1987.

249. Otsuji S, Shibata H, Umeda M. Turbidimetric immunoassay of serum C-reactive protein. Clin Chemi. 1982;28(10):2121-4.

250. Guevara I, Iwanejko J, Dembińska-Kieć A, Pankiewicz J, Wanat A, Anna P, et al. Determination of nitrite/nitrate in human biological material by the simple Griess reaction. Clin Chim Acta. 1998;274(2):177-88.

251. Ohkawa H, Ohishi N, Yagi K. Assay for lipid peroxides in animal tissues by thiobarbituric acid reaction. Anal Biochem. 1979;95(2):351-8.

252. Richardson RJ, Murphy SD. Effect of glutathione depletion on tissue deposition of methylmercury in rats. Toxicol Appl Pharmacol. 1975;31(3):505-19.

253. Lowry OH, Rosebrough NJ, Farr AL, Randall RJ. Protein measurement with the Folin phenol reagent. J Biol Chem. 1951;193(1):265-75.

254. Leslie E, Geoffrey J, James M. Statistical analysis. Interpretation and uses of medical statistics. 4th ed: Oxford Scientific Publications (pub); 1991. p. 411-6.

255. Armitage A. Statistical methods in medical research. Oxoford and Edinburgh. Blackwell Scientific Publications; 1999. p. 99-146.

256. Puri BK. SPSS in Practice: An Illustrated Guide. Arnold: London; 2002. p. 320.

257. Palsamy P, Sivakumar S, Subramanian S. Resveratrol attenuates hyperglycemia-mediated oxidative stress, proinflammatory cytokines and protects hepatocytes ultrastructure in streptozotocin-nicotinamide-induced experimental diabetic rats. Chem Biol Interact. 2010;186(2):200-10.

258. Kamenova P. Improvement of insulin sensitivity in patients with type 2 diabetes mellitus after oral administration of alpha-lipoic acid. Hormones (Athens). 2006;5(4):251-8.

259. Petersen KF, Shulman GI. Pathogenesis of skeletal muscle insulin resistance in type 2 diabetes mellitus. Am J Cardiol. 2002;90(5A):G11-8.

260. Lenzen S, Drinkgern J, Tiedge M. Low antioxidant enzyme gene expression in pancreatic islets compared with various other mouse tissues. Free Radic Biol Med. 1996;20(3):463-6.

261. Erejuwa OO, Sulaiman SA, Wahab MS, Salam SK, Salleh MS, Gurtu S. Antioxidant protective effect of glibenclamide and metformin in

combination with honey in pancreas of streptozotocin-induced diabetic rats. Int J Mol Sci. 2010;11(5):2056-66.

262. Xu H, Barnes GT, Yang Q, Tan G, Yang D, Chou CJ, et al. Chronic inflammation in fat plays a crucial role in the development of obesity-related insulin resistance. J Clin Invest. 2003;112(12):1821-30.

263. Wellen KE, Hotamisligil GS. Inflammation, stress, and diabetes. J Clin Invest. 2005;115(5):1111-9.

264. Staels B, Fruchart JC. Therapeutic roles of peroxisome proliferator-activated receptor agonists. Diabetes. 2005;54(8):2460-70.

265. Jensen MD. Adipose tissue as an endocrine organ: implications of its distribution on free fatty acid metabolism. Eur Heart J Suppl. 2006;8(suppl B):B13-9.

266. Gual P, Le Marchand-Brustel Y, Tanti JF. Positive and negative regulation of insulin signaling through IRS-1 phosphorylation. Biochimie. 2005;87(1):99-109.

267. Zhang M, Lv XY, Li J, Xu ZG, Chen L. The characterization of high-fat diet and multiple low-dose streptozotocin induced type 2 diabetes rat model. Exp Diabetes Res. 2008;2008:704045.

268. Srinivasan K, Viswanad B, Asrat L, Kaul CL, Ramarao P. Combination of high-fat diet-fed and low-dose streptozotocin-treated rat: a model for type 2 diabetes and pharmacological screening. Pharmacol Res. 2005;52(4):313-20.

269. Dresner A, Laurent D, Marcucci M, Griffin ME, Dufour S, Cline GW, et al. Effects of free fatty acids on glucose transport and IRS-1-associated phosphatidylinositol 3-kinase activity. J Clin Invest. 1999;103(2):253-9.

270. Ahmed OM, Mahmoud AM, Abdel-Moneim A, Ashour MB. Antihyperglycemic and antihyperlipidemic effects of hesperidin and naringin in high fat diet/streptozotocin type 2 diabetic rats. Life Sci J. 2011;8(4):91-101.

271. Sahin K, Onderci M, Tuzcu M, Ustundag B, Cikim G, Ozercan IH, et al. Effect of chromium on carbohydrate and lipid metabolism in a rat

model of type 2 diabetes mellitus: the fat-fed, streptozotocin-treated rat. Metabolism. 2007;56(9):1233-40.

272. Zhang Z, Xue HL, Liu Y, Wang WJ. Yi-Qi-Zeng-Min-Tang, a chinese medicine, ameliorates insulin resistance in type 2 diabetic rats. World J Gastroenterol. 2011;17(8):987-95.

273. Ojiako OA, Nwanjo HU. Effects of pioglitazone on atherogenic risk predictor indices of alloxan-induced diabetic rabbits. J Biochem. 2005;17(2):179-84.

274. Vijayaraghavan K. Treatment of dyslipidemia in patients with type 2 diabetes. Lipids Health Dis. 2010;9(144):1-12.

275. Al-Rawi NH. Oxidative stress, antioxidant status and lipid profile in the saliva of type 2 diabetics. Diab Vasc Dis Res. 2011;8(1):22-8.

276. Avramoglu RK, Basciano H, Adeli K. Lipid and lipoprotein dysregulation in insulin resistant states. Clin Chim Acta. 2006;368(1-2):1-19.

277. Watanabe M, Houten SM, Wang L, Moschetta A, Mangelsdorf DJ, Heyman RA, et al. Bile acids lower triglyceride levels via a pathway involving FXR, SHP, and SREBP-1c. J Clin Invest. 2004;113(10):1408-18.

278. Iwasaki T, Takahashi S, Takahashi M, Zenimaru Y, Kujiraoka T, Ishihara M, et al. Deficiency of the very low-density lipoprotein (VLDL) receptors in streptozotocin-induced diabetic rats: insulin dependency of the VLDL receptor. Endocrinology. 2005;146(8):3286-94.

279. Wang HJ, Jin YX, Shen W, Neng J, Wu T, Li YJ, et al. Low dose streptozotocin (STZ) combined with high energy intake can effectively induce type 2 diabetes through altering the related gene expression. Asia Pac J Clin Nutr. 2007;16(1):412-7.

280. Feingold KR, Lear SR, Moser AH. De novo cholesterol synthesis in three different animal models of diabetes. Diabetologia. 1984;26(3):234-9.

281. Wu CH, Lin JA, Hsieh WC, Yen GC. Low-density-lipoprotein (LDL)-bound flavonoids increase the resistance of LDL to oxidation

and glycation under pathophysiological concentrations of glucose in vitro. J Agric Food Chem. 2009;57(11):5058-64.

282. Kalogerakis G, Baker AM, Christov S, Rowley KG, Dwyer K, Winterbourn C, et al. Oxidative stress and high-density lipoprotein function in Type I diabetes and end-stage renal disease. Clin Sci (Lond). 2005;108(6):497-506.

283. Hussein Ael -A, Omar NM, Sakr H, Elsamanoudy AZ, Shaheen D. Modulation of metabolic and cardiac dysfunctions by insulin sensitizers and angiotensin receptor blocker in rat model of type 2 diabetes mellitus. Can J Physiol Pharmacol. 2011;89(3):216-26.

284. Lewis GF, Carpentier A, Adeli K, Giacca A. Disordered fat storage and mobilization in the pathogenesis of insulin resistance and type 2 diabetes. Endocr Rev. 2002;23(2):201-29.

285. Peters AL. Clinical relevance of non-HDL cholesterol in patients with diabetes. Clin Diabetes. 2008;26(1):3-7.

286. Bittner V, Johnson BD, Zineh I, Rogers WJ, Vido D, Marroquin OC, et al. The triglyceride/high-density lipoprotein cholesterol ratio predicts all-cause mortality in women with suspected myocardial ischemia: a report from the Women's Ischemia Syndrome Evaluation (WISE). Am Heart J. 2009;157(3):548-55.

287. Parveen K, Khan R, Siddiqui WA. Antidiabetic effects afforded by Terminalia arjuna in high fat-fed and streptozotocin-induced type 2 diabetic rats. Int J Diabetes & Metab. 2011;19:23-33.

288. Ohtsuki T, Matsumoto M, Suzuki K, Taniguchi N, Kamada T. Mitochondrial lipid peroxidation and superoxide dismutase in rat hypertensive target organs. Am J Physiol. 1995;268(4 Pt 2):H1418-21.

289. Kumawat M, Pahwa MB, Gahlaut VS, Singh N. Status of antioxidant enzymes and lipid peroxidation in type 2 diabetes mellitus with micro vascular complications. Open Endocrinol J. 2009;3:12-5.

290. Parveen K, Khan M, Mujeeb M, Siddiqui WA. Protective effects of Pycnogenol on hyperglycemia-induced oxidative damage in the liver of type 2 diabetic rats. Chem Biol Interact. 2010;186(2):219-27.

291. Nourooz-Zadeh J, Rahimi A, Tajaddini-Sarmadi J, Tritschler H, Rosen P, Halliwell B, et al. Relationships between plasma measures of oxidative stress and metabolic control in NIDDM. Diabetologia. 1997;40(6):647-53.

292. Seghrouchni I, Drai J, Bannier E, Rivière J, Calmard P, Garcia I, et al. Oxidative stress parameters in type I, type II and insulin-treated type 2 diabetes mellitus; insulin treatment efficiency. Clin Chim Acta. 2002;321(1-2):89-96.

293. Scott JA, King GL. Oxidative stress and antioxidant treatment in diabetes. Ann N Y Acad Sci. 2004;1031(1):204-13.

294. Choi SW, Benzie IFF, Ma SW, Strain JJ, Hannigan BM. Acute hyperglycemia and oxidative stress: direct cause and effect? Free Radic Biol Med. 2008;44(7):1217-31.

295. Rasilainen S, Nieminen JM, Levonen AL, Otonkoski T, Lapatto R. Dose-dependent cysteine-mediated protection of insulin-producing cells from damage by hydrogen peroxide. Biochem Pharmacol. 2002;63(7):1297-304.

296. Livingstone C, Davis J. Review: Targeting therapeutics against glutathione depletion in diabetes and its complications. Br J Diabetes Vasc Dis. 2007;7(6):258-65.

297. Paolisso G, Giugliano D. Oxidative stress and insulin action: is there a relationship? Diabetologia. 1996;39(3):357-63.

298. Davis BJ, Xie Z, Viollet B, Zou MH. Activation of the AMP-activated kinase by antidiabetes drug metformin stimulates nitric oxide synthesis in vivo by promoting the association of heat shock protein 90 and endothelial nitric oxide synthase. Diabetes. 2006;55(2):496-505.

299. de Luca C, Olefsky JM. Inflammation and insulin resistance. FEBS Lett. 2008;582(1):97-105.

300. Tam CS, Viardot A, Clément K, Tordjman J, Tonks K, Greenfield JR, et al. Short-term overfeeding may induce peripheral insulin resistance without altering subcutaneous adipose tissue macrophages in humans. Diabetes. 2010;59(9):2164-70.

301. Sena CM, Matafome P, Louro T, Nunes E, Fernandes R, Seiça RM. Metformin restores endothelial function in aorta of diabetic rats. Br J Pharmacol. 2011;163(2):424-37.

302. Amin KA, Awad EM, Nagy MA. Effects of panax quinquefolium on streptozotocin-induced diabetic rats: role of C-peptide, nitric oxide and oxidative stress. Int J Clin Exp Med. 2011;4(2):136-47.

303. Wang C, Li J, Lv X, Zhang M, Song Y, Chen L, et al. Ameliorative effect of berberine on endothelial dysfunction in diabetic rats induced by high-fat diet and streptozotocin. Eur J Pharmacol. 2009;620(1-3):131-7.

304. Pickup JC. Inflammation and activated innate immunity in the pathogenesis of type 2 diabetes. Diabetes care. 2004;27(3):813-23.

305. Dandona P, Aljada A, Bandyopadhyay A. Inflammation: the link between insulin resistance, obesity and diabetes. Trends Immunol. 2004;25(1):4-7.

306. El-Osta A, Brasacchio D, Yao D, Pocai A, Jones PL, Roeder RG, et al. Transient high glucose causes persistent epigenetic changes and altered gene expression during subsequent normoglycemia. J Exp Med. 2008;205(10):2409-17.

307. van den Oever IA RH, Nurmohamed MT, Simsek S. Endothelial dysfunction, inflammation, and apoptosis in diabetes mellitus. Mediators Inflamm. 2010;2010(792393):1-15.

308. Schalkwijk CG, Stehouwer CD. Vascular complications in diabetes mellitus: the role of endothelial dysfunction. Clin Sci (Lond). 2005;109(2):143-59.

309. Hayden MR, Tyagi SC. Intimal redox stress: accelerated atherosclerosis in metabolic syndrome and type 2 diabetes mellitus. Atheroscleropathy. Cardiovasc Diabetol. 2002;1(1):1-27.

310. Zahedi Asl S, Ghasemi A, Azizi F. Serum nitric oxide metabolites in subjects with metabolic syndrome. Clin Biochem. 2008;41(16-17):1342-7.

311. Matsumoto T, Noguchi E, Ishida K, Kobayashi T, Yamada N, Kamata K. Metformin normalizes endothelial function by suppressing vasoconstrictor prostanoids in mesenteric arteries from OLETF rats, a model of type 2 diabetes. Am J Physiol Heart Circ Physiol. 2008;295(3):H1165-76.

312. Salpeter SR, Buckley NS, Kahn JA, Salpeter EE. Meta-analysis: metformin treatment in persons at risk for diabetes mellitus. Am J Med. 2008;121(2):149-57.e2.

313. El-Batran SA, Abdel-Salam OM, Nofal SM, Baiuomy AR. Effect of rosiglitazone and nateglinide on serum glucose and lipid profile alone or in combination with the biguanide metformin in diabetic rats. Pharmacol Res. 2006;53(1):69-74.

314. Foretz M, Hébrard S, Leclerc J, Zarrinpashneh E, Soty M, Mithieux G, et al. Metformin inhibits hepatic gluconeogenesis in mice independently of the LKB1/AMPK pathway via a decrease in hepatic energy state. J Clin Invest. 2010;120(7):2355-69.

315. Moreno-Navarrete JM, Ortega FJ, Rodríguez-Hermosa JI, Sabater M, Pardo G, Ricart W, et al. OCT1 expression in adipocytes could contribute to increased metformin action in obese subjects. Diabetes. 2011;60(1):168-76.

316. Steiner CA, Janez A, Jensterle M, Reisinger K, Forst T, Pfützner A. Impact of treatment with rosiglitazone or metformin on biomarkers for insulin resistance and metabolic syndrome in patients with polycystic ovary syndrome. J Diabetes Sci Technol. 2007;1(2):211-7.

317. Domieh AM, Khajehlandi A. Effect of 8 weeks endurance training on plasma visfatin in middle-aged men. Braz J Biomotricity. 2010;4(3):174-9.

318. Wulffelé MG, Kooy A, de Zeeuw D, Stehouwer CDA, Gansevoort RT. The effect of metformin on blood pressure, plasma cholesterol

and triglycerides in type 2 diabetes mellitus: a systematic review. J Intern Med. 2004;256(1):1-14.

319. Ginsberg H, Plutzky J, Sobel BE. A review of metabolic and cardiovascular effects of oral antidiabetic agents: beyond glucose-level lowering. J Cardiovasc Risk. 1999;6(5):337-46.

320. Yki-Järvinen H, Ryysy L, Nikkilä K, Tulokas T, Vanamo R, Heikkilä M. Comparison of bedtime insulin regimens in patients with type 2 diabetes mellitus. A randomized, controlled trial. Ann Intern Med. 1999;130(5):389-96.

321. Robinson AC, Burke J, Robinson S, Johnston DG, Elkeles RS. The effects of metformin on glycemic control and serum lipids in insulin-treated NIDDM patients with suboptimal metabolic control. Diabetes Care. 1998;21(5):701-5.

322. Groop L, Widén E, Franssila-Kallunki A, Ekstrand A, Saloranta C, Schalin C, et al. Different effects of insulin and oral antidiabetic agents on glucose and energy metabolism in type 2 (non-insulin-dependent) diabetes mellitus. Diabetologia. 1989;32(8):599-605.

323. Rains SG, Wilson GA, Richmond W, Elkeles RS. The effect of glibenclamide and metformin on serum lipoproteins in type 2 diabetes. Diabet Med. 1988;5(7):653-8.

324. DeFronzo RA, Goodman AM. Efficacy of metformin in patients with non-insulin-dependent diabetes mellitus. The Multicenter Metformin Study Group. N Engl J Med. 1995;333(9):541-9.

325. Wulffelé MG, Kooy A, Lehert P, Bets D, Ogterop JC, Borger van der Burg B, et al. Combination of insulin and metformin in the treatment of type 2 diabetes. Diabetes Care. 2002;25(12):2133-40.

326. Lund SS, Tarnow L, Frandsen M, Smidt UM, Pedersen O, Parving HH, et al. Impact of metformin versus the prandial insulin secretagogue, repaglinide, on fasting and postprandial glucose and lipid responses in non-obese patients with type 2 diabetes. Eur J Endocrinol. 2008;158(1):35-46.

327. Tiikkainen M, Häkkinen AM, Korsheninnikova E, Nyman T, Mäkimattila S, Yki-Järvinen H. Effects of rosiglitazone and metformin on liver fat content, hepatic insulin resistance, insulin clearance, and gene expression in adipose tissue in patients with type 2 diabetes. Diabetes. 2004;53(8):2169-76.

328. Rabbani N, Chittari MV, Bodmer CW, Zehnder D, Ceriello A, Thornalley PJ. Increased glycation and oxidative damage to apolipoprotein B100 of LDL cholesterol in patients with type 2 diabetes and effect of metformin. Diabetes. 2010;59(4):1038-45.

329. Zhou G, Myers R, Li Y, Chen Y, Shen X, Fenyk-Melody J, et al. Role of AMP-activated protein kinase in mechanism of metformin action. J Clin Invest. 2001;108(8):1167-74.

330. Musi N, Hirshman MF, Nygren J, Svanfeldt M, Bavenholm P, Rooyackers O, et al. Metformin increases AMP-activated protein kinase activity in skeletal muscle of subjects with type 2 diabetes. Diabetes. 2002;51(7):2074-81.

331. Viollet B, Foretz M, Guigas B, Horman S, Dentin R, Bertrand L, et al. Activation of AMP-activated protein kinase in the liver: a new strategy for the management of metabolic hepatic disorders. J Physiol. 2006;574(Pt 1):41-53.

332. Giorgino F, Laviola L, Leonardini A. Pathophysiology of type 2 diabetes: rationale for different oral antidiabetic treatment strategies. Diabetes Res Clin Pract. 2005;68(1):S22-9.

333. Ghatak SB, Dhamecha PS, Bhadada SV, Panchal SJ. Investigation of the potential effects of metformin on atherothrombotic risk factors in hyperlipidemic rats. Eur J Pharmacol. 2011;659(2-3):213-23.

334. Hoeger K, Davidson K, Kochman L, Cherry T, Kopin L, Guzick DS. The impact of metformin, oral contraceptives, and lifestyle modification on polycystic ovary syndrome in obese adolescent women in two randomized, placebo-controlled clinical trials. J Clin Endocrinol Metab. 2008;93(11):4299-306.

335. Zhang XF, Tan BK. Antihyperglycaemic and anti-oxidant properties of Andrographis paniculata in normal and diabetic rats. Clin Exp Pharmacol Physiol. 2000;27(5-6):358-63.

336. Pavlović D, Kocić R, Kocić G, Jevtović T, Radenković S, Mikić D, et al. Effect of four-week metformin treatment on plasma and erythrocyte antioxidative defense enzymes in newly diagnosed obese patients with type 2 diabetes. Diabetes Obes Metab. 2000;2(4):251-6.

337. Kumar PV, Ramesh N, Bricey AA, Selvi VV. Evaluation of lipid peroxidation and antioxidants activity of metformin in high fructose fed diet induced type II diabetic rats. IJPT. 2010;2(3):456-64.

338. Tripathi UN, Chandra D. Diabetes induced oxidative stress: A comparative study on protective role of Momordica charantia and metformin. Phcog Res. 2009;1(5):299-306.

339. Hou X, Song J, Li XN, Zhang L, Wang XL, Chen L, et al. Metformin reduces intracellular reactive oxygen species levels by upregulating expression of the antioxidant thioredoxin via the AMPK-FOXO3 pathway. Biochem Biophys Res Commun. 2010;396(2):199-205.

340. Marchetti P, Del Guerra S, Marselli L, Lupi R, Masini M, Pollera M, et al. Pancreatic islets from type 2 diabetic patients have functional defects and increased apoptosis that are ameliorated by metformin. J Clin Endocrinol Metab. 2004;89(11):5535-41.

341. Rösen P, Wiernsperger NF. Metformin delays the manifestation of diabetes and vascular dysfunction in Goto-Kakizaki rats by reduction of mitochondrial oxidative stress. Diabetes Metab Res Rev. 2006;22(4):323-30.

342. United Kingdom Prospective Diabetes Study (UKPDS) Group. Effect of intensive blood-glucose control with metformin on complications in overweight patients with type 2 diabetes. Lancet. 1998;352(9131):854-65.

343. Ouslimani N, Mahrouf M, Peynet J, Bonnefont-Rousselot D, Cosson C, Legrand A, et al. Metformin reduces endothelial cell expression of both the receptor for advanced glycation end products and lectin-like oxidized receptor 1. Metabolism. 2007;56(3):308-13.

344. Mithieux G, Guignot L, Bordet JC, Wiernsperger N. Intrahepatic mechanisms underlying the effect of metformin in decreasing basal glucose production in rats fed a high-fat diet. Diabetes. 2002;51(1):139-43.

345. Arai M, Uchiba M, Komura H, Mizuochi Y, Harada N, Okajima K. Metformin, an antidiabetic agent, suppresses the production of tumor necrosis factor and tissue factor by inhibiting early growth response factor-1 expression in human monocytes in vitro. J Pharmacol Exp Ther. 2010;334(1):206-13.

346. Isoda K, Young JL, Zirlik A, MacFarlane LA, Tsuboi N, Gerdes N, et al. Metformin inhibits proinflammatory responses and nuclear factor-κB in human vascular wall cells. Arterioscler Thromb Vasc Biol. 2006;26(3):611-7.

347. Hattori Y, Suzuki K, Hattori S, Kasai K. Metformin inhibits cytokine-induced nuclear factor κB activation via AMP-activated protein kinase activation in vascular endothelial cells. Hypertension. 2006;47(6):1183-8.

348. Bruun JM, Lihn AS, Pedersen SB, Richelsen B. Monocyte chemoattractant protein-1 release is higher in visceral than subcutaneous human adipose tissue (AT): implication of macrophages resident in the AT. J Clin Endocrinol Metab. 2005;90(4):2282-9.

349. Dandona P. Effects of antidiabetic and antihyperlipidemic agents on C-reactive protein. Mayo Clin Proc. 2008;83(3):333-42.

350. Haffner S, Temprosa M, Crandall J, Fowler S, Goldberg R, Horton E, et al. Intensive lifestyle intervention or metformin on inflammation and coagulation in participants with impaired glucose tolerance. Diabetes. 2005;54(5):1566-72.

351. Caballero AE, Delgado A, Aguilar-Salinas CA, Herrera AN, Castillo JL, Cabrera T, et al. The differential effects of metformin on markers of endothelial activation and inflammation in subjects with impaired glucose tolerance: a placebo-controlled, randomized clinical trial. J Clin Endocrinol Metab. 2004;89(8):3943-8.

352. Pilon G, Dallaire P, Marette A. Inhibition of inducible nitric-oxide synthase by activators of AMP-activated protein kinase: a new mechanism of action of insulin-sensitizing drugs. J Biol Chem. 2004;279(20):20767-74.

353. Tesseraud S, Métayer Coustard S, Collin A, Seiliez I. Role of sulfur amino acids in controlling nutrient metabolism and cell functions: implications for nutrition. Br J Nutr. 2009;101(8):1132-9.

354. Diniz YS, Rocha KK, Souza GA, Galhardi CM, Ebaid GM, Rodrigues HG, et al. Effects of N-acetylcysteine on sucrose-rich diet-induced hyperglycaemia, dyslipidemia and oxidative stress in rats. Eur J Pharmacol. 2006;543(1-3):151-7.

355. Kinscherf R, Cafaltzis K, Röder F, Hildebrandt W, Edler L, Deigner HP, et al. Cholesterol levels linked to abnormal plasma thiol concentrations and thiol/disulfide redox status in hyperlipidemic subjects. Free Radic Biol Med. 2003;35(10):1286-92.

356. El-Bassiouni EA, Helmy MH, El-Zoghby SM, El-Nabi KM, Hosny RM. Relationship between level of circulating modified LDL and the extent of coronary artery disease in type 2 diabetic patients. Br J Biomed Sci. 2007;64(3):109-16.

357. Parthimos T, Tsopanakis C, Angelogianni P, Schulpis KH, Parthimos N, Tsakiris S. L-cysteine supplementation prevents exercise-induced alterations in human erythrocyte membrane acetylcholinesterase and Na+, K+-ATPase activities. Clin Chem Lab Med. 2007;45(1):67-72.

358. Cheng X, Xia Z, Leo JM, Pang CC. The effect of N-acetylcysteine on cardiac contractility to dobutamine in rats with streptozotocin-induced diabetes. Eur J Pharmacol. 2005;519(1-2):118-26.

359. Souza GA, Ebaid GX, Seiva FR, Rocha KH, Galhardi CM, Mani F, et al. N-Acetylcysteine an Allium plant compound improves high-sucrose diet-induced obesity and related effects. Evid Based Complement Alternat Med. 2008:Epub ahead of print.

360. Stanislaus R, Gilg AG, Singh AK, Singh I. N-acetyl-L-cysteine ameliorates the inflammatory disease process in experimental

autoimmune encephalomyelitis in Lewis rats. J Autoimmune Dis. 2005;2(1):1-11.

361. Ho E, Chen G, Bray TM. Supplementation of N-acetylcysteine inhibits NFκB activation and protects against alloxan-induced diabetes in CD-1 mice. FASEB J. 1999;13(13):1845-54.

362. Ramasamy S, Drummond GR, Ahn J, Storek M, Pohl J, Parthasarathy S, et al. Modulation of expression of endothelial nitric oxide synthase by nordihydroguaiaretic acid, a phenolic antioxidant in cultured endothelial cells. Mol Pharmacol. 1999;56(1):116-23.

363. Pieper GM, Siebeneich W. Oral administration of the antioxidant, N-acetylcysteine, abrogates diabetes-induced endothelial dysfunction. J Cardiovasc Pharmacol. 1998;32(1):101-5.